THE MEDITERRANEAN
DIET FOR BEGINNERS

Discover the Secrets to Lose Weight in Just 30 Days. Diet With a Meal Plan and Simple, Easy, and Healthy Recipes. Enjoy Your Food Every Day.

Alexander Phenix

© Copyright 2020 - All rights reserved.

from various sources. Please consult a licensed professional before attempting any techniques outlined in this book.

By reading this document, the reader agrees that under no circumstances is the author responsible for any losses, direct or indirect, that are incurred as a result of the use of the information contained within this document, including, but not limited to, errors, omissions, or inaccuracies.

Table of Contents

Introduction

Up until recently there was little known about how major health conditions affected the rest of the world. You have probably assumed, like so many others, that the leading cause of death in America has to be the same in other countries around the world. Though the U.S. is one of the wealthiest countries, our bill of health doesn't match up with many of the other countries around the world.

Our fast-paced life, convenient means of travel, and quick stop meals has taken a major toll on our health and happiness. Millions of Americans are suffering from unpaid medical bills, countless prescription drugs, and debilitating health conditions. There is so much finger-pointing at what the cause is that many are neglecting to see that the problem is right in front of them and so is the solution.

Heart disease, diabetes, obesity, and mental health issues are on the rise in America and around the world. While many factors can contribute to each of these detriments, poor diet is the leading factor causing all these problems. So few people are aware of the impact diet plays in obtaining and maintaining optimal health. And many more seem to blatantly ignore the serious side effects that their poor food choices are causing them

Food doesn't just affect your waistline. It doesn't just help your heart and body function properly. The foods you eat can also have a significant impact on your mood and mental health. When you have a combination of a poor diet that coincides with excessive stress, and little to no physical activity, the hormones, and neurotransmitters in your brain are not firing off the happy feel-good chemical that keeps you happy.

High-fat, excess sodium, sugar-loaded, and low nutrient foods are the go-to choice for every meal of the day. We live in a time where everything has to be quick and easy. The solution comes in the form of highly processed and prepackaged foods sold for convenience and nothing else. Convenience didn't put health as a priority, instead, it made quick and easy, available for busy families to eat and go. It made sitting down to eat a healthy meal something that was a burden and presented a solution that caused increased health problems and a decrease in mealtime socialization. You shouldn't have to sacrifice health for convenience but this is what many of us are taught. As a result, we are overweight, sleep-deprived, and heading for a shorter life filled with medical issues.

The quick-fix solution was to combat the long list of health issues with new diets and food trends arising regularly. These diets make promises of rapid weight loss. But, rarely are these fad diets teaching you how to actually maintain a long-term healthy lifestyle. Instead of turning to food as a form of medicine or preventive measure to reduce serious health risks, we look at healthy options as a form of punishment.

We go on diet after diet trying to regain our energy and perfect body image only to fall back into the same patterns that lead us there, to begin with. We choose convenience over health. Many times this convenience is not really convenient in terms of saving time or money, and especially not when it comes to your health.

Sticking to a diet is never easy. Having to eat the same foods every day that are often bland and unsatisfying is no way to maintain a healthy life. But dieting is not the long term answer. Jumping on the next fad diet bandwagon isn't going to prevent you from falling into the same habits and thought patterns that revolve around the food you eat. For years you have looked at healthy foods as an inconvenience and this isn't going to be a quick thought pattern to change. Jumping into a quick fix diet may give you the result you seek but they won't be long-lasting.

Instead, create a new healthy lifestyle. When you begin to look at food as a nourishing form of medicine and not as a quick way to combat hunger pains you will begin to make healthier choices.

If you have tried countless diets, then you might have felt like there was no way that you could stick to the diet for the long term because the food was bland and boring. Being healthy shouldn't result in sacrificing flavor and satisfaction. If your food doesn't taste good you won't stick to the diet, no matter how beneficial it is to your health. Instead, being able to enjoy your food because it tastes good and is beneficial to your health will result in making healthy eating a lifestyle.

The problem with many diets that seem to pop up every year is that they are unsustainable. They can be expensive and are not meant to be followed for an extended period of time. What tends to occur is you go from dieting back to your normal diet, and as a result, see a return of health problems and weight gain.

Many diets focus on cutting out specific food groups or sticking to a restrictive diet that is bland and unmotivating. The problem with this is, cutting out specific food groups when sticking to these diets means cutting out specific nutrients your body needs to function properly.

The Mediterranean diet is not just about eating healthy, it is about living a healthy lifestyle. Exercise and coming together to share a nutritious meal is vital. This diet is about learning to form a better relationship with food while also incorporating healthy activities to improve your overall health.

The Mediterranean Diet Pyramid, which you will learn more about in this book, is an effective tool that will assist you in transitioning to this healthier lifestyle. It incorporates not just foods to eat but activities to include in your daily life. The Mediterranean Diet Pyramid will change the way you create meals and look at your lifestyle as a whole.

The Mediterranean diet has been followed by the Greeks, Italians and other populations located around the Mediterranean Sea. The people in this are showing a lower number of reporter health issues like diabetes, heart disease, and obesity. Compared to the American population, which follows a Western Diet, the individuals in these regions were significantly more healthy and happy. They are reported to have a much lower risk of major illnesses that are leading to death in the United States.

Researchers took notice of the significant difference in health status between the Americans and those residing in Italy and Greece. Studies have been and continue to look out how the Mediterranean Diet and Western diet affects the health of those on it. What has been proven is that those following the Mediterranean diet had much better health, and when individuals switched from their Western diet to the Mediterranean diet, their health improved. The Mediterranean diet has been shown to reduce the risk of heart attack, stroke, and premature death while also preventing the development of conditions such as Type 2 diabetes.

The Mediterranean Diet is recognized by UNESCO as the cultural heritage of Greece, Italy, Morocco, and Spain (Rockbridge Press, 2013). This interchangeable way of living served as a model lifestyle that promoted not only optimal health in these regions and surrounding areas but served as a guideline for individuals to live a longer and happier life. Additionally, the Mediterranean diet has been considered the best diet for overall health as well as from those suffering from heart conditions, diabetes, and cognitive decline (Rockbridge Press, 2013).

It is also considered to be one of the easiest diets to follow to significantly improve your health. And, yet so few are following it. We have grown into the habit of thinking prepacked and convenient is easier than fresh and wholesome. We have been taught to think that making a nutritious home-cooked meal takes hours of time out of our already busy schedule. In reality, making meals that adhere to the Mediterranean diet takes just as much time, and sometimes less, as unwrapping your store-bought dinner and popping it into the oven. What we are taking as convenience now from prepacked and process we will suffer from later in hospital bills, medications, and less satisfying life.

The information provided to you in this book will not only give you a better understanding of what the Mediterranean diet is, but you will also learn how to transition from an unhealthy diet to the Mediterranean diet with ease. You will find an easy to follow reference guide that will reveal the steps to take to transition to the Mediterranean diet gradually. You will also find it easy to follow recipes that you can begin using today to start living a more healthy life. The recipes will prove to you that health doesn't have to be hard and you can make it conveniently work for your busy schedule and life.

The simple changes to your lifestyle discussed in this book will increase your longevity and reduce your risk of mental and physical health issues. It will help you rewire the way you think about the word "diet". It will open your eyes to a whole new lifestyle that not only focuses on improving your eating habits but increasing physical activity and making connections with those around you.

The Mediterranean diet focuses on healthy and delicious foods. If you have been struggling to adhere to a more healthy way of eating, want to be able to cut out the processed and pre-packaged foods from your diet, and want to stress less about your health, then the Mediterranean diet is your solution. This inexpensive diet is satisfying and easy to follow.

It is time for you to let go of the misconceptions you have carried about health and learn to change your perspective. The Mediterranean diet can be the solution to your health concerns, lack of energy, and mental health troubles. If you are ready to have more energy and better overall health, without having to sacrifice flavorful and delicious meals, then read on. You will learn that healthy meals don't have to be boring and that health is more than just the foods you eat, it is an entire lifestyle.

Chapter 1:
What is the Mediterranean Diet?

The term diet often leads one to think of having to count calories, restrict foods, and can cause a mindset of deprivation. A low-carb diet, the Atkins diet, Ketogenic diet, and many other diets, were formulated to result in rapid weight loss by cutting out foods that actually have nutritional value. That is what makes these diets so appealing. While maintaining a healthy weight is an important aspect of living a healthy life, the focus should not be on strictly losing weight. A diet should be something that you can make a part of your lifestyle. This is why so many individuals who begin these different types of fad diets may see great success in losing weight quickly, but when they transition back to their normal eating habits, that weight is gained back just as quickly.

A diet needs to be sustainable. It needs to be something that does take much thought and becomes a habit. The Mediterranean diet is not about restricting food and does not focus on cutting or tracking calories. Many individuals who follow the Mediterranean diet guidelines will often eat without concern about taking in too many calories. The Mediterranean diet goal is to help you successfully eliminate the unhealthy foods you consume and replace them with whole foods. The Greek word *diaita* for diet translates to means a way of living (CulinaryLore, 2018). It is not just the food and beverages you consume but the habits, activities, and people you fill your life with.

The Mediterranean diet is a sustainable lifestyle that allows you to live a healthy and satisfying life. It emphasizes enjoying seasonal and fresh locally grown fruits and vegetables. Whole grains, healthy fats, legumes, beans, and fish make up a majority of the rest of the diet. Food groups such as dairy and red meats are still enjoyed just not to the extent that the Western Diet tends to. Dairy is limited to a few small servings a week while red meat is included just once or twice a month.

It is not a research created diet though it is a diet that has been thoroughly researched. The Mediterranean diet does not try to get you to restrict foods but instead, encourages whole nutritious foods that can become a way of life. It is based on the lifestyle of those living in the specific countries of the Mediterranean. It's an easy to follow the way of planning your meals that is inspired by the way individuals would eat in the 1950s and 1960s in the Mediterranean areas. For the people living there, pre-packaged and processed foods were not readily available. Most of the people in these areas were not wealthy and grew much of their own fruits and vegetables. They used the fresh produce they had on hand and included small portions of fish or poultry occasionally. They focused on creating flavorful plant-based meals that could be easily shared and enjoyed by neighbors, family, and friends.

You may see a difference in food choices depending on which region you look at. Some regions incorporate a great deal more legumes and lentils while others may enjoy more whole grain options. The similarity, however, is that all these regions enjoy plenty of plant-based foods and limit or completely eliminate processed and prepackaged foods as well as added sugars and refined foods from their diets. Each region consumes nearly 2 to 3 times as many fruits and vegetables as those on a Western diet, and enjoy healthy fats like olive oil, nuts, and seeds regularly.

There isn't much thought for people in these areas when it comes to planning their meals. Eating more nutrient-rich foods like fresh fruits and vegetables is such an ingrained way of life for them that they rarely stress over whether they are eating a healthy diet or not.

A Typical Mediterranean Diet Consists of:

1. Fresh produce like organic fruits and vegetables make up a majority of the diet.

2. A variety of whole grains like barley, millet, and whole wheat are enjoyed frequently but usually as side dishes.

3. Legumes, lentils, and beans are included in most meals each day of the week. These foods tend to make up a significant source of protein since there is limited consumption of red meats

4. Healthy fats such as unrefined olive oil, nuts, and seeds are consumed daily.

5. Fish and other kinds of seafood are incorporated into weekly meals at least twice a week.

6. Small portions of poultry like chicken, turkey, or duck are enjoyed a few times a week.

7. Red meats are lean and grass-fed and enjoyed on special occasions and usually one once or twice a month.

8. Red wine is included in moderation, and it is not uncommon for a glass of red wine to be enjoyed a day.

Mealtimes Are a Social Event

What makes the Mediterranean diet so unique is it transforms mealtimes into an experience. The dining room table is a place to gather and socialize. Meals are seen as a time to relax and reconnect with family and friends.

In the western world, many are used to making meals as quickly as possible. Meals are often approached as an obligation instead of a time to slow down. It is not uncommon for many American tables to have family members sitting around glued to the phones scrolling social media and watching YouTube. This is not connecting. This is disconnecting but a disconnect from the wrong things. When you put down the phones, turn off the TV, and enjoy the company of those around you you actually reduce stress and will notice a boost to your mood.

Aside from the stress release and mood increase, eating with others often reduces your risk of overeating. This is also a vital time that you can connect and support your children while also instilling healthy eating habits within your children.

It isn't just the eating that is a social experience. Preparing meals is also made into social events. It is not uncommon to have multiple people in the kitchen helping out and sharing their days and the latest news. When others are invited over for dinner they are encouraged to come earlier to participate in the preparations. Some even do the grocery shopping together. This allows individuals to deepen their connection and stay connected.

Physical Activity

Partaking in physical activity is just a part of daily life for those in the Mediterranean. This is partially due to the ease of walking safely, everything located nearby, and a culture of walking. But, aside for these factors, these individuals choose to just walk to the store, family house, or a friend's house. This regular physical activity also plays a major role in exceptional health.

Most individuals who follow the Mediterranean diet also get about 2 ½ hours of cardio or aerobic exercise a week. This is often divided up throughout the week and is squeezed in doing typical daily chores. Yard work, cleaning the house, vacuuming, working in your garden or even enjoying time running and dancing around with your kids are simple ways that you can get in a little bit of aerobic exercise in 10-minute intervals.

Some exercises to consider:

- Cycling

- Jogging

- Swimming

- Yoga

- HIIT

- Running

- Walking

- Resistance training

- Strength training

30-Minutes Workout Sample

This simple exercise routine can be done anywhere. There are 5 different moves that you will do a certain number of times. Once you complete all 5 moves you will take a short break and then repeat the whole sequence for a total of three times. You can easily add in additional moves and swap in different moves when you feel the need to change things up. Before you begin this workout, be sure to properly warm up your body. Do a few jumping jacks, run in place, stretch your arms and legs, and twist your torso. You don't want to injure yourself, even if you feel the workout is relatively easy it might not take much for you to tear a muscle or suffer from some form of injury. The same is true when you are done with the workout. Take a few minutes to cool down by doing a number of stretches like touching your toes, calf stretches, and arm stretches.

- 20 Standard squats

- 10 Push-ups

- 10 Lunges on each leg

- 20 Jumping jacks

- 20-Second plank

Feel free to utilize this workout routine 2 to 3 days a week to help break up your exercise routine. Remember, exercise should be something you enjoy so choose something that works for you and that you know you will keep going back to. You can also make physical activity a family activity. Enjoy running outside with your kids or dancing around in the living room. This will help them start living a Mediterranean lifestyle from a young age so they can benefit from having optimal health for the rest of their lives.

Chapter 2:
Where Did the Mediterranean Diet Come From?

The Mediterranean diet is inspired by the eating habits of the populations that surround the Mediterranean Sea. The populations of southern Italy and Greece are the main regions that influence this diet. But, it isn't the diet that is consumed today in many of these regions that gained so much attention. The Mediterranean diet refers to the traditional eating habits and lifestyles of these areas in the 1950s and 1960s. It was during this time that researchers noticed a significant difference in the health of populations in these areas when compared to those living in America. It was obvious that many of the individuals in the Mediterranean areas were healthier and the key difference between those living in the Mediterranean and those living in America was their diet.

Ancel Keys

Though it has always been evident that the diet of those residing in the Mediterranean regions was healthy, there was little scientific data to make the connections between their lifestyle and better health. Ancel Keys was a physiologist who spent a great deal of his career studying dietary patterns and the effects they had on a person's health. He was one of the first researchers to take a closer look at why the individuals living in the Mediterranean region had much better heart health than those living in the United States.

Ancel Keys was incredibly meticulous in his research when it came to finding a connection between diet and heart disease. He believed that saturated fats could be the key culprit that would increase the risk of individuals suffering from coronary heart disease. In 1958, he was able to launch what is referred to as the "Seven Country Study" (Rockridge Press, 2013). This study closely examined the dietary habits of those residing in Finland, Greece, Italy, Japan, South Africa, Spain, and the United States. Though the data provided from the study included seven countries, a total of 16 cohorts were conducted to partake in the research. There was no financial support to aid in the study which took place over a 10-year span. Each of the countries that agreed to participate in the long-term study did so by using their own funding, which in the 1960s was a challenge for many countries after the series of wars and struggles most faced.

What he discovered from this study was a significantly lower rate of coronary heart disease among even the poorest populations in these areas compared to the population of America. This was true even when he closely looked at the wealthy individuals in America, who were believed to be healthy simply because they could afford to be. It wasn't just the Americans who were suffering from an increase in heart disease. Finland reported the second-highest number of individuals with heart disease. When the diets of the American groups and the Finland group were examined they uncovered that each consumed a diet high in saturated fats and animal fats. Whereas the countries with the lowest reports of heart disease consumed a diet that was made up of mostly fresh vegetables, whole grains, fish, and unsaturated fats.

His findings were some of the first to indicate that heart disease and the risk of a heart attack could be prevented. Since then a number of studies have been conducted to take a closer look at why those in the Mediterranean seemed to be living healthier and happier lives.

The Harvard School of Public Health along with the Athens Medical School in Greece conducted a study in 2003 that indicated those following a Mediterranean diet had longer lifespans (Rockridge Press, 2013). Another study in 2008, focused on how the Mediterranean diet could help individuals lose weight (Rockridge Press, 2013). Even more striking is that in America, those who follow a Mediterranean diet have significantly lowered their risk of not just heart disease, but also cognitive decline, diabetes, and mental health issues (Rockridge Press, 2013). Research continues today that shows how eating a diet that is rich in fresh fruits, vegetables, healthy fat, and whole grains, like the Mediterranean diet, can improve one's health drastically. There are hundreds of case studies and research data that has shown how switching to a Mediterranean diet can reduce the risk of heart disease, considered to be the leading cause of death in America. It has been shown to reduce the effect of diabetes and help prevent cognitive decline.

Despite all the evidence that points out the undeniable benefits of the Mediterranean diet, not everyone is quick to follow the Mediterranean diet. In fact, individuals living in the Mediterranean today, do not even follow the traditional way of life that made the area one of the healthiest in the world just a few decades ago.

There is a great deal of debate about some of the components of the Mediterranean diet that twist the facts. Eating healthy fats is one of the most attacked aspects of the Mediterranean diet. For a while all fats were looked at as bad because there was little understanding of the various forms of fats the body could use for energy, this is also true of carbohydrates. What Ancel Keys discovered, as well as many other researchers, was that the fats consumed with the Mediterranean diet are ones that differed greatly from the fats being consumed in excess in the United States. It was actually healthy fats like olive oil that was one of the biggest contributors to the optimal health of individuals of the time.

Another misconception was red meat. People believed that cutting out red meat from one's diet was unhealthy. Red meat was supposed to be one of the only forms of protein you could eat and eating red meat only occasionally was the opposite of what the United States Department of Agriculture was suggesting.

The Food Pyramid vs. The Mediterranean Diet Pyramid

The food pyramid serves as a standard guideline for what a healthy well-balanced diet should look like. It was created by the United States Department of Agriculture (USDA) so individuals could better follow and understand recommended food servings. The USDA food pyramid offered Americans an easy to follow a template of what they should eat daily.

This food pyramid has been under continual attack, and there were several other versions that were released before the most well-known version was made public in the 1990s. Each of the previous versions was criticized by food companies stating it would cause the general public to stop buying their products (Roycor, A., and Roycor, A., 2017). It seems as though the food pyramid that was created was not one that took the health of the people in the United States into consideration but was more of a marketing stunt for food companies.

At the bottom of the USDA pyramid, you will find the grains food group with the recommendation of 6 to 11 servings a day. This group includes bread, pasta, rice, and cereals. Above the grains are the fruits and vegetables. Fruits have a recommendation of 2 to 4 servings a day while these vegetables have a recommendation of 3 to 6 servings.

Next up on the pyramid is a line that divides up the dairy and meat food groups. Dairy is recommended to be consumed 2 to 3 times a day. The meat group, which includes red meats, poultry, fish, beans, eggs, and nuts recommends that you eat 2 to 3 servings a day. At the very top of the pyramid, you'll find the "use sparingly" category. In this category, you'll find the oils, sweets, and fats.

While this pyramid may have been helpful for food manufacturers to boost sales, there is a great deal of controversy around it. The fact that it has not specified which types of grains should be consumed or that healthy fats and unhealthy fats are grouped together are the first discrepancies. The other is the daily recommendations are out of balance. According to this pyramid, your diet should consist of mostly grains.

Recently, a newer design of the pyramid is being used. Instead of a pyramid, it uses a plate to show individuals how much each food group should fill their plates at each meal. While there is a noticeable difference in portion size, vegetables seem to fill more of the plate than the other food groups. Fats are often completely left out of the diagram.

To combat the original USDA food pyramid, the Mediterranean food pyramid came about. The Mediterranean diet pyramid was created with the help of the Harvard School of Public Health and the World Health Organization (WHO) (Oldway's Mediterranean Diet Pyramid, n.d.). It showed foods displayed in the same pyramid formation but it didn't include daily recommendations for all of the food groups and further divided groups in affordances to their health benefits. The foods at the bottom of the list should be consumed on a daily basis. The foods in the middle of the pyramid should be consumed a few times a week. And foods at the top of the pyramid should be consumed on a monthly basis.

According to the Mediterranean diet pyramid, extra virgin olive oil and other healthy fats like nuts and seeds along with whole grains, fruits, vegetables, legumes, and beans sit at the bottom of the pyramid. Above this large section, you will find the fish and seafood group. Next is poultry, eggs, cheese, and nonfat dairy. At the very top of the pyramid is the red meat and sweets group. There are some significant differences between the USDA food pyramid and the Mediterranean diet pyramid

First, the USDA grouped all meat together on the pyramid. There is no distinction made between whether you should eat more red meat or fish for better overall health.

The Mediterranean diet clearly emphasized fruits, vegetables, and healthy fats to be consumed on a daily basis. It also made physical activities and connecting with others a priority. No other diet took into consideration the importance of these last two factors. While everyone suggests exercising for losing weight it is rarely suggested as part of a diet plan to live a long healthy life.

It is argued that the Mediterranean diet is not an ideal diet for most people around the world to adapt to. As you continue to read, you will learn just how simple it is to begin transitioning to a Mediterranean diet. You will see that all the food groups included in the Mediterranean diet are easily available no matter where you live.

Chapter 3:
What Do You Eat on the Mediterranean Diet?

The Mediterranean diet focuses on including as many plant-based foods into your diet as possible. The diet consists primarily of fresh vegetables, fruits, and healthy oils. Legumes, whole grains, and fish are also included in many meals. Dairy, poultry, and red meats are consumed less frequently though not entirely eliminated from the diet. With this diet, you will be eating more of what your body needs and therefore, will crave less of the unhealthy foods that you have grown accustomed to. In this chapter, we will cover the core food groups that make up the Mediterranean diet as well as the other types of foods you can include.

Vegetables

Fresh vegetables make up a majority of the Mediterranean diet. They are often eaten raw or slightly cooked to preserve the vitamins and nutrients. Bitter greens, such as kale, broccoli rabe, spinach, and chard, are some of the most nutritious vegetables you can include in your diet. They are loaded with an array of vitamins such as vitamins A, C, and K. Many bitter greens also provide you with a healthy dose of omega-3 fatty acids and are an excellent source of fiber and folate. They can help aid and stimulate digestion and rid the body of toxins. These dark leafy vegetables are available in many varieties all through the year. They are easy to incorporate into your diet and you should aim to have at least one serving of bitter greens a day.

Aside from daily serving of bitter greens you want your meals to be primarily vegetables. Those living in the Mediterranean regions tend to eat over three times the number of servings of vegetables than most Americans. Most meals, like lunch and dinner, tend to consist of only vegetables and only sometimes will they include a small portion of meat. Most dinners, which will often be a variety of roasted, steamed, or stew vegetables will also be accompanied by salads or other raw vegetable dishes.

When it comes to choosing your vegetables it is best to go with locally farmed organic varieties. These will deliver the maximum amount of nutrition. Farmer markets in the spring, summer, and fall months will provide you with some of the best organically grown vegetables. This follows the Mediterranean example of eating locally grown foods. If you do not have access to local farmer markets in your area look for organic vegetables in your local grocery store. Nowadays, most grocery stores dedicate a wide section to organically grown produce so you will find a nice variety to pick from. Keep in mind, most fresh organic vegetables can be frozen and saved for later. So never worry about buying too much of a certain item.

If organic is not an option, you can still choose raw produce. Many large companies own farms that supply stores with these vegetables. They use chemicals to treat their crops which get absorbed into the plant and make its way to your dinner plate. When buying these types of fresh vegetables be sure to thoroughly wash and sometimes scrub the outside of the vegetable before consuming.

Frozen vegetables are another way for you to stock up on a variety of vegetables. You may not get as much of the vitamins and nutrients with frozen vegetables but they are still a good choice when looking for easy ways to include more veggies into your diet.

Vegetables sold in cans should be avoided if possible. Though they are an incredibly cheap way to quickly add in vegetables, they offer significantly fewer nutrients and are often loaded with sodium and other preservatives. Also keep in mind, that after sitting for an extended amount of time in the canning package it is possible for the vegetables stored in the can to begin to absorb some of the properties from the can. This can cause you to consume an even higher amount of harmful chemicals that can cause serious health problems over time. You don't want to swap out the health benefits you get from fresh produce just for the convenience of opening a can and reheating the contents. Plus, canned vegetables will most often have a less desirable taste than fresh produce.

When choosing your vegetables choose a wide variety. Be adventurous and include something new into your weekly meal plan. Vegetables come in all colors and including a little bit from each color group will provide you with a balance of minerals, vitamins, and nutrients.

Fruits

Like vegetables, the Mediterranean diet encourages fruit to be consumed regularly. Fruits are enjoyed for breakfast, snacks, and will often be served after dinner as a dessert. Fresh organic fruits are the best options and can be frozen to use in smoothies, ice cream, and more.

Many Mediterranean recipes will also include a number of citrus fruits into their recipes. Lemon is one of the most popular fruits used in Mediterranean cooking and lemon wedges are plentiful around the dinner table. But, you don't have to stick with the fruits that many people in this area are accustomed to eating. The Mediterranean diet is about eating the fresh foods that are locally and seasonally available where you reside.

Healthy Oils and Fats

The first thing many people will tell you to cut out from your diet is excess fat. What they don't tell you is that not all fats are the same. Healthy fats consist of unsaturated fats like monounsaturated fat or polyunsaturated fats. These fats can help boost your health because they help with digestion, assist the body in absorbing nutrients, can help you feel full and are important for heart and brain health.

Olive oil is a kitchen staple in Mediterranean countries, but the olive oil consumed in Mediterranean areas is quite different from the oil found in many American homes. You can taste the differences from the olive oil typically used in the United States. Olive oil in the U.S. typically has a light or inoffensive taste. However, in Mediterranean countries, olive oil is flavorful and rich in taste.

Extra virgin olive oil refers to the oil that comes from the first press of the olives. The oil is extracted through a cold-press process that requires no chemicals and preserves the most nutrients and flavor. This oil is rich in antioxidants, is thicker and unfiltered, which is why it has many many health benefits. Unfiltered extra virgin olive oil has a distinct peppery taste. This causes a slight burn if consumed raw which is due to the anti-inflammatory properties.

Aside from olive oil, the Mediterranean diet includes plenty of nuts and seeds. Almonds, walnuts, Brazilian nuts, and chia seeds are some nuts and seeds that are sources of healthy fats. They can also provide you with protein, magnesium, and vitamin E. Eating a moderate amount of various nuts and seeds can help keep blood pressure low, reduce the risk of chronic diseases, and prevent heart disease and diabetes.

Legumes

Legumes tend to be consumed at least once a day on the Mediterranean diet. Legumes take the place of meat on the Mediterranean diet. For many Mediterranean populations, lentils are consumed more frequently than you find in America because many regions fast during religious holidays for extended periods of time. During these fasting times, they refrain from eating any and all animal products. Beans are an easy replacement. Since fasting tends to take place for a large portion of the year,

Mediterraneans simply stick with their diet of mainly consuming beans instead of meat.

Beans are highly popular and range in flavor. Chickpeas, garbanzo beans, lentils, and white beans are some of the most commonly used beans in the Mediterranean and are easily found in bulk in the United States. They are quite easy to cook, despite what many think. They are also not as time-consuming. Though many beans need to be pre-soaked before cooking to soften them, this can often be done overnight.

Canned beans are an easy alternative to dried beans. But they should be drained and rinsed to remove the excess sodium. Cooking dry beans is not as challenging or a time-consuming process as many think. Though dried beans do need to be soaked for eight or more hours, this doesn't require you to do much except put them in a bowl and cover with water. After they are done soaking they can be drained and used in any meal.

Whole Grains

Bread, rice, pasta, and other grains are a staple in the Mediterranean diet. There tends to always be a basket of bread served with lunch and dinner for everyone to share. But, you won't necessarily find white bread on the tables. Most of the bread consumed on the Mediterranean diet tends to be sourdough, or at least is made with a sourdough starter as opposed to the yeast starters used with the bread consumed by many Americans.

Barley and wheat are the most used grains in Mediterranean meals. Grains do not make up a majority of the meals on the Mediterranean diet. Large plates or bowls of pasta are not typical. Instead, whole grains will be served as a small side dish and will always be accompanied by vegetables, olive oil, or beans.

Fish

Many think the Mediterranean diet is closely related to a pescatarian diet, where fish is the most consumed animal product. While a variety of seafood is consumed on the Mediterranean diet, it is often only included in meals two or three times a week. The portions are also fairly small, especially when compared to standard American servings. Anchovies, sardines, and wild-caught fatty fish make up a majority of the fish consumption. Fish also serves as a healthy form of fat on the Mediterranean diet, which is why it is in its own category and separated from red meats.

Other seafood items like octopus and scallops are shared around the dinner table. They are often not breaded or fried as you have probably had them prepared. They instead are grilled and drizzled with olive oil and lemon juice.

Fish is often served simply with olive oil, capers, and lemon. You will find fish soups and stews are very popular in the Mediterranean region. Portions are kept small and always served with plenty of vegetables. There are many ways you can enjoy fish on the Mediterranean diet and you don't have to stick with the fish that are available locally in that region. Many areas in the United States don't have the luxury of enjoying freshly caught fish, but you can still enjoy this healthy item when you look for frozen fish.

Some people avoid eating fish because of the high traces of mercury that is found in some species. While this is a concern, for the most part, larger types of fish like swordfish, shark, and tuna tend to have the highest amount of mercury. Most of the fish used in Mediterranean cooking has very low levels of mercury. This low level of mercury along with the limited consumption does not pose a health risk to those who eat it.

Dairy

Dairy is not excluded from the Mediterranean diet but it is consumed in moderation. Dairy products, especially milk, tend to have a high amount of saturated fats which can increase blood pressure, clogged arteries, and have serious negative effects on your health. Instead of eliminating dairy, the Mediterranean diet encourages nonfat dairy options. Many regions that inspired the Mediterranean diet enjoy feta cheese, yogurt, ricotta, and parmesan cheese. Low-fat or nonfat options are favored and necessary for bone and heart health. It is not common for many to drink milk on the Mediterranean diet and instead will choose water over milk.

Poultry

Free-range chicken, turkey, duck, and organic eggs are consumed regularly on the Mediterranean diet, though not as much as they tend to be consumed with a Western diet. These items are often consumed a few times a week. They are prepared by roasting and rarely ever bread and fried as many enjoy it prepared on the Western diet. When poultry is included in a meal, it tends to be a small portion to complement the rest of the meal, not take the spotlight of the meal.

Red Meat

When it comes to consuming red meat, the Mediterranean diet keeps consumption to a minimum. Often red meat is only consumed once or twice a month or only on special occasions. It tends to serve as a side dish instead of the main ingredient. Fish, poultry, and beans are used in place of red meats during most meals.

When red meat is consumed, grass-fed, organic meats are highly recommended. Grass-fed animals tend to be healthier and produce much leaner cuts of meat. When choosing red meats to eat while adopting the Mediterranean diet, choose lean cuts that are 90 percent lean with 10 percent fat.

Chapter 4:
What Foods Are Not Allowed on the Mediterranean Diet?

The Mediterranean diet does not outwardly restrict foods but, it does emphasize the importance of replacing well-known unhealthy items with more healthy options. This will help you transition from a more Western diet to a Mediterranean diet with more success. When you begin to think that you can't have something while on a diet, you begin to have a craving. You tend to crave that item more and you are more likely to overindulge on the item you are told you can't have. Shift your mindset from focusing on what you are not eating to what you are eating. Fresh fruits can be just as satisfying as an ice cream sundae but are much more healthy for you. Crispy fresh vegetables can replace chips and provide you with the same crunchy textures. Though you are not required to eliminate the following items, if you want to truly experience all of the benefits of the Mediterranean diet and not only lose weight but improve your overall health it is strongly suggested you do. To make it easier we have not only covered what items you could avoid but also a simple way to replace them with healthier options.

Added Sugar

Sugar will probably be the most difficult item to cut from your diet as it is simple in just about everything you buy. When you begin to remove buying pre-packaged and processed foods and buy more fruits and vegetables a lot of added sugar will just naturally fall out of your diet. Sugar is added to many food items and not just snack foods and sodas. Added sugar can be found in pasta sauces, peanut butter, fruit juices, bread products, and many processed foods. These sugars are considered empty calories and often contain different chemicals. Some of the most commonly added sugars you might be familiar with include:

- High fructose corn syrup
- Glucose
- Corn syrup
- Sucrose
- Maltose
- Corn sweetener

Those who struggle with weight loss often do not consider the exuberant amount of sugar they are consuming because they are often a hidden ingredient. Added sugar can make it more difficult for you to stop eating. When you consume an excessive amount of fructose your body is unable to produce leptin. Leptin is the hormone that is released to signal your body that you are full. It is necessary for you to regulate when you need to eat and when you need to stop. This often leads to eating more food than you need and consuming high amounts of calories.

What to replace them with?

- Eat fresh fruits when you have a sweet craving.

- Replace sugar-filled drinks like soda and fruit juices with water. You can add fresh fruit pieces like strawberries and raspberries to give your water more flavor.

- Instead of using refined sugars switch to organic sweeteners like pure organic honey or maple syrup.

Refined Grains

Refined grains have been linked to a number of serious health conditions such as Type 2 diabetes and heart disease. The misunderstanding about grains is that they all get grouped in with carbohydrates and many view carbs as bad. But while not all carbs are bad, this isn't the case when we are talking about refined grains. Refined grains have gone through a milling process to remove the bran and germ from the grain. When the process is complete you are left with a fine-textured grain that has a long shelf life. What this also does is remove a majority of the nutrients from the grain. There is little fiber, iron, and vitamins that remain in the grains after they have been milled.

What you are left with is a high-calorie food that offers no nutrition. The most common refined grains consist of:

- White flour
- White bread
- White rice
- White flour pizza crust
- Breakfast cereals

Though some of these products will be enriched with some of the vitamins and that were originally stripped during the milling process, the fiber and other nutrients are not added back in. Keep in mind that even enriched refined grains have preservatives and additives to give the products more flavor and to last longer.

Whole grains are a much better alternative but you need to be aware that even whole grain products may be a mixture of refined grains and whole grains. Always check the food labels to be sure of what you are buying. If you catch the word enriched anywhere on the label then it is a mixture of whole and refined grains.

What to replace them with?

- Choose sourdough bread when possible.

- Enjoy sandwiches in a whole grain wrap or pita bread.

- Try plant-based alternatives like cauliflower crust, cauliflower rice, or spiralized vegetables in place of pasta.

- Swap in whole grains like quinoa and brown rice.

Refined Oils

Refined oils are incredibly damaging to your health. These types of oils are not only refined, meaning most of the key nutrients have been stripped from the product, but additional chemicals have been used in the process. These chemicals remain in the oil and end up making their way to your kitchen.

When oils are refined, they are often treated with acid or go through a purifying process that involves alkali. Some oils will be neutralized, filtered, or deodorized using additional chemicals. This process allows manufacturers to extract the most oil out of the seeds.

Most oils are extracted from the seeds of plants; this can include soybean oil, corn oil, sunflower oil, peanut oil, and olive oil. Vegetable oils are a combination of multiple parts of plants. The process of extracting the oil involves a variety of chemicals that can increase inflammation in the body. The fat that remains in the oil has been linked to a number of health conditions such as cancer, heart disease, and diabetes.

Oils are also used to create margarine in a hydrogenation process. This process uses chemicals that will allow the oil to remain in a solid-state. When the oil is hydrogenated, the fatty acids that were in the oil are further destroyed and transformed into trans fatty acids. A number of scientific studies have been conducted to show trans fatty acid's connection to a number of debilitating health conditions. Trans fatty acids are considered to be some of the most unhealthy fats you can consume, especially when it comes to your heart. These industrially manufactured fats cause LDL cholesterol to increase. High amounts of LDL or bad cholesterol can clog and destroy your arteries and increase blood pressure. This significantly increases your risk of heart attack and stroke.

The most consumed refined oils are partially hydrogenated vegetable oils. This is because they are much cheaper and are a common ingredient in prepackaged and processed foods. Unfortunately, food manufacturers do not have to clearly specify whether or not their product contains hydrogenated oils or trans fats. This means you can read the food label and think you are safe but can actually consume a large quantity of these harmful oils. This is why it is best to avoid or at least significantly reduce your intake of processed foods.

Some of the most common items that contain trans fats or hydrogenated oils that you might not be aware of include:

- Microwaveable popcorn

- Butter

- Margarine

- Vegetable oil

- Fried foods or fast foods

- Pre-packaged muffins, cakes, doughnuts, and pastries.

- Coffee creamers

- Prepared pizza dough or pizza crust

- Cake frosting

- Potato chips

- Crackers

The Mediterranean diet focuses on replacing these refined oils and processed foods with more wholesome and natural ingredients.

What to replace them with?

- Refined oils can be easy to eliminate from your diet. If you are used to sautéing your foods with refined oil such as butter or margarine, switch to unrefined olive oil.

- Instead of frying foods in oil, bake them in the oven or grill them on an outside grill or using a grill pan.

- Invest in a quality set of non-stick pots and pans. This way you only have to add a little bit of water to the skillet or pot and won't have to worry about it sticking.

- Enjoy avocado on toast instead of butter.

Processed Meat

Processed meats are a number of meats that have been processed extensively to preserve flavors and provide a longer shelf life. The most common types of processed meats include bacon, hot dogs, pre-packaged lunch or deli meats, sausage, and canned meats.

A number of studies have shown the link between the consumption of processed meats and an increased risk of cancer, heart disease, and diabetes. The International Agency for Research on Cancer (IARC) categorized processed meat as a Group 1 carcinogen. This puts it in the same cancer-causing category as asbestos and tobacco (Are processed red meats, 2019). Studies show that consuming processed meat daily can cause or increase the risk of colorectal cancer, stomach cancer, pancreatic cancer, and prostate cancer (Are processed red meats, 2019). There has also been a direct link in an increase of coronary heart disease and an increased risk of diabetes in individuals who consumed some form of processed meat on a daily basis. This can be as little as one hot dog or a few slices of deli meat.

Processed meats tend to contain the same amount of saturated fat and cholesterol as unprocessed red meats. What makes processed meats so harmful is the amount of sodium found in these products. Processed meats contain over four times the amount of sodium than red meats. Sodium is already known to increase blood pressure which increases the risk of different heart diseases.

The preservatives found in processed meat are another factor that causes a decline in health. Processed meat contains at least 50% more preservatives than unprocessed meats. These preservatives affect sugar tolerances and can cause insulin resistance that can lead to diabetes.

What to replace them with?

- Switch out processed meats and red meats for fish or poultry.

- Use vegetables or beans in place of meat.

- Use a variety of spices to add more flavor to a dish where you would use meat in the same way. Spices like cumin, coriander, peppercorn, and marjoram add unique flavors to the dish so you won't miss the bacon, sausage, or ground meat. You can use different seasonings on sauteed or baked vegetables.

- Use roasted chickpeas or toasted seeds and nuts to dishes for more texture. These can be great alternatives to dishes that call for bacon crumbles.

Chapter 5:
Myths and Facts of the Mediterranean Diet

There are always going to be rumors and negative perspectives on any type of "diet" that gets put in the spotlight. The Mediterranean diet is no exception. There are a number of questions that people ask and assumptions made when one begins to consider the Mediterranean diet. Most of these myths and misinformation come from simply not having a clear understanding of what the Mediterranean diet really is. Here we will dig deeper into the most common myths, misconceptions, and facts that will help you decide if this is the way of life that can truly benefit you.

Myth 1: The Mediterranean Diet is Expensive

The Mediterranean diet consists of mostly plant-based foods. Beans, lentils, and many fresh vegetables cost significantly less than buying packaged dinners. You can spread your ingredients out over various meals. A dozen eggs can serve you breakfast and be incorporated into dinner recipes. Fresh vegetables are used in every meal so you never have to worry about them going to waste. Buying from the farmers market also cuts down the cost of eating fresh organic fruits and vegetables.

When compared to the cost of eating a Western diet, the Mediterranean diet is far less expensive. One fast-food meal on the Western diet can equal three or four meals on the Mediterranean diet. In the long term, having a clean bill of health will cost far less in medical expenses. The Western diet not only costs more upfront but will cost you thousands due to poor health in the future.

Myth 2: Mediterraneans Drink Red Wine in Large Quantities, so Drinking Hard Liquor Should be Fine

One to two glasses of red wine can provide health benefits. The antioxidants in red wine are beneficial for your heart health. Drinking an excessive amount of red wine though can have negative effects on your health. Hard liquor is not encouraged on the Mediterranean diet either. Hard liquor in any amount can increase your risk of certain cancers. When consumed in excess, long term drinking can cause serious damage to your heart, liver, and brain health. Beer is also not recommended as it usually contains a significant number of calories that can lead to adding on pounds and becoming overweight.

Myth 3: The Mediterranean Diet Encourages Large Servings of Pasta and Breads

This myth may have to do with the fact that parts of Italy are considered part of the Mediterranean region and parts of Italy have been closely researched because of their healthy lifestyles. Though pasta is considered a traditional and unrestricted dish for Italians, the Mediterraneans approach pasta differently. Instead of pasta is the highlight of the meal it tends to be served as a side dish. This is true for bread as well. Bread is always served but is offered with olive oil and olives for dipping.

Myth 4: The Mediterranean Diet is Just Like Any Other Diet; it Only Focuses on the Food You Eat

As it has been stressed throughout this book, the Mediterranean diet is not just about eating the right foods. The Mediterraneans get plenty of physical activity through walking, cycling, or hiking. While eating a diet rich in organic fruits and vegetables is important there is more to the diet than just what you eat. How you eat is also an important aspect. Unlike most individuals who eat a Western diet, Mediterraneans sit down to enjoy food and relax with their family while they are eating. It is a very rare occurrence that you will see households in front of the television while eating a meal or grabbing their food to go. Sharing home-cooked meals and socializing is important and contributes to their overall happiness.

Myth 5: The Mediterranean Diet Cannot be Followed Outside of the Mediterranean

The guidelines for the Mediterranean diet can be followed by anyone living anywhere in the world. In fact, many populations have transitioned to this diet because of the many health benefits. The Mediterranean diet includes eating more locally grown and seasonal fruits and vegetables, not just eating the fruits and vegetables available in the Mediterranean regions. No matter where you live you can easily begin to include more fruits and vegetables that are plentiful in your area. Most of the foods of the Mediterranean are easily found in North America and other countries. Tomatoes, for example, are common vegetables eaten in the Mediterranean that you can find just about anywhere all year round. Additionally, there are some foods that are not local to the Mediterranean that can be easily included in your diet and still adhere to the Mediterranean diet.

For example, blueberries and apples are more readily available in the United States then they are in the Mediterranean. This diet is not specific about which fruits and vegetables or whole grain you need to consume. It is incredibly flexible with these main components so that just about anyone can benefit from following a more Mediterranean diet.

Myth 6: The Mediterranean Diet is a High-Fat Diet

Olive oil, nuts, seeds, and avocados do contain a high amount of fat. And these items are enjoyed frequently on the Mediterranean diet. It can be considered a high-fat diet when you look at it in terms of the high-fat content in the foods you are eating. But, unlike other high-fat foods, the focus is on consuming quality fats. The fats you eat on the Mediterranean diet are packed with antioxidants, are good for your health, and can help reduce the risk of many health issues. While technically you can look at it as a high-fat diet, this is not comparable to the high-fat diets consumed in the United States and some other countries around the world. Many other high-fat diets do not take into consideration where the fat comes from or what type of fats is being consumed. This often results in consuming high amounts of saturated and trans fats. The fats on the Mediterranean diet are polyunsaturated fats or monounsaturated fats.

Myth 7: The Mediterranean Diet is Not Something You Can Follow For a Long Time

The Mediterranean diet, at a glance, can seem like a complex eating plan. But really it is about swapping out unhealthy choices with more healthy ones. The only thing that makes this diet seem as though it cannot be adhered to for the long-term is the fact that you will have to get used to eating in a different way and for a different reason. For years you have eaten and prepared your meals a certain way. When you begin on the Mediterranean diet, it can feel overwhelming because you aren't used to this way of eating or preparing meals. But, just as you have learned how to walk, read, and pay your own bills, the more you do it, the easier it becomes. The Mediterranean is not complex but the way we have been taught to think about preparing whole foods is that it is time-consuming and hard. Once you have been on it for a few weeks and begin to notice a change in your energy, sleep, mood, and health it becomes easier.

Myth 8: You Won't Lose Weight on the Mediterranean Diet

If you are overweight or obese, there is a good chance you will lose a significant amount of weight on the Mediterranean diet. Even if you are only looking to lose a few pounds, the Mediterranean diet can help you lose weight and keep it off. Though it is not and has never been a fad diet for weight loss, when you begin to eat more healthy foods and include physical activity into your daily routine, you will notice extra weight come off. If you are trying to lose weight on the Mediterranean diet, and plan to continue with this diet even after you have lost the weight, you can simply reduce your calorie intake by 300-500 calories a day. If you are just trying to lose weight fast, this isn't the diet for you.

Myth 9: But People in the Mediterranean Eat Plenty of Junk Food

It is true, the diet of those living in the Mediterranean regions today includes a number of items that the Mediterranean diet tries to avoid. Those in the area today eat more junk food, processed foods, and sugars. And over the last decade or two, there has been a significant increase in reported coronary heart disease, cancers, and other serious health concerns that were nearly non-existent in the region when research on the Mediterranean diet first began. What we call the Mediterranean diet is actually the diet of the region 70 years ago in the 1950s and '60s. Unfortunately, today this traditional way of enjoying food is not as strongly followed in the region and the decline in this population's health reflects that.

Myth 10: Following the Mediterranean Diet Means You Can Eat Much Bigger Meals

When you begin the Mediterranean diet, it might seem like you are eating significantly more food. For some, this might be true. The difference between the Mediterranean diet and the Western diet that many are accustomed to is portion size and types of foods consumed. Those on the Mediterranean diet can eat more than those following a Western diet if you look at the number of calories consumed. Most Western meals are oversized and packed with calories and little nutrients. You can easily consume more than half the recommended calorie intake for the day with just one meal on a Western diet. Mediterranean meals tend to be smaller, or they will have a variety of foods offered in smaller portions. They also tend to snack on healthy foods throughout the day, but the meals are packed with nutrients. You may start your meal off with a simple salad, followed by the main course that is mostly vegetables and sometimes a small piece of fish, poultry, or red meat will accompany the vegetarian main course but won't take up your dinner plate. Beans or whole grains will also be served as a side dish or a small amount will be included in the main dish. Additional vegetables will be offered up on the side as well. This sounds like a never-ending flow of food and it can look that way but in reality, all this food adds up to few calories and substantial nutrients. Many of the fruits and vegetables they consume contain very little calories so they can, in fact, eat more. When it comes to vegetables and fruits, you can eat as much as you like, everything else is in moderation. So while you may be able to eat more on the Mediterranean diet, you are eating more of the healthy foods, cooked with healthy oils, and served with good company.

Chapter 6:
What are the Benefits
of a Mediterranean Diet?

The Mediterranean diet gained popularity in the medical fields because of its documented benefits to heart health. But, plenty of research has shown that the Mediterranean diet can have a much longer list of health benefits that go beyond the heart. This chapter will go over just a few of the many improvements you can experience with your health when you start on the Mediterranean diet.

Heart Health and Reduced Risk of Stroke

The Mediterranean diet first gained attention because of the significantly low numbers of reported coronary heart disease in the regions of the Mediterranean. There are many components of the Mediterranean diet that help promote heart health. By reducing and eventually eliminating your consumption of processed foods, refined grains, and processed meats you reduce your risk of a number of heart conditions including heart attack and stroke. The diet focuses on replacing unhealthy trans fats with healthier unsaturated or monounsaturated fats. Fresh fish, fruits, and vegetables that are high in fiber, omega-3 fatty acids, and antioxidants are consumed daily.

Heart health is greatly impacted by diet. Maintaining healthy levels of good cholesterol, blood pressure, blood sugar, and staying within a healthy weight results in optimal heart health. Your diet directly affects each of these components. Those who are at greater risk are often advised to begin adhering to a low-fat diet. A low-fat diet cuts out all fats including those from oils, nuts, and red meats. Studies have shown that the Mediterranean diet, which includes healthy fats, is more effective at lowering cardiovascular risks than a standard low-fat diet (Are processed red meats, 2019). This is because the unsaturated fats consumed on the Mediterranean diet not only lower bad cholesterol levels, but also increase good cholesterol levels.

The Mediterranean diet also stresses the importance of daily activity and stress reduction by enjoying quality time with friends and family. Each of these elements, along with eating more plant-based foods, significantly improves heart health and reduces the risk of many heart-related conditions. By increasing your intake of fresh fruits and vegetables while adding in regular daily activities, you improve not just your heart health but overall health.

Reduces Age-Related Muscle and Bone Weakness

Eating a well-balanced diet that provides you with a wide range of vitamins and minerals is essential for reducing muscle weakness and bone degradation. This is especially important as you age. Accident related injuries such as tripping, falling or slipping while walking can cause serious injury. As you age, this becomes even more of a concern as some simple falls can be fatal. Many accidents occur because of weakening muscle mass and the loss of bone density. Women, especially those who are entering the menopause phase of their life, are at a greater risk of serious injury from accidental falls because the estrogen levels decline significantly at this time. This decrease in estrogen results in a loss of bone and muscle mass. The decrease of estrogen can also cause bone-thinning which over time develops into osteoporosis.

Maintaining healthy bone mass and muscle agility as you age can be challenging. When you are not getting the proper nutrients to promote healthy bones and muscles, you increase your risk of developing osteoporosis. The Mediterranean diet offers you a simple way to fulfill the dietary needs necessary to improve bone and muscle functioning.

Antioxidants, vitamins C and K, carotenoids, magnesium, potassium, and phytoestrogens are essential minerals and nutrients for optimal musculoskeletal health. Plant-based foods, unsaturated fats, and whole grains help provide you with the necessary balance of nutrients that keep your bones and muscles healthy. Sticking with a Mediterranean diet can improve and reduce the loss of bone mass as you age.

Reduces the Risk of Alzheimer's

Alzheimer's disease is a form of dementia where there is significant cognitive decline. Those with Alzheimer's suffer from:

- Disorientation
- Memory Loss
- Inability to think clearly
- Speech problems
- Impaired judgment
- Visual and spatial disorientation

Alzheimer's is a common brain disorder in older adults, 60 years of age or older, but the first signs of Alzheimer's can be present in adults as young as 30 years of age. The condition can progress fast or slowly depending on how quickly the neurons in the brain begin to die off. Though the decline begins in the hippocampus area of the brain it becomes widespread as it progresses.

Individuals with Alzheimer's show a significant increase in beta-amyloid proteins in the brain and have a much lower level of brain energy. Research has focused on trying to identify those who are at greater risk of dementia early on through brain scans and imaging. In one such study, brain scans were conducted on 70 individuals between the ages of 30 and 60. None of the participants showed signs of dementia and 34 of them adhered to a Mediterranean diet while 36 followed a standard Western diet. When brain scans were conducted at the beginning of the study and then two years later. The scans showed that those on the Western diet had significant loss in brain energy levels and an increase in the beta-amyloid build-up as opposed to those on the Mediterranean diet (Mediterranean Diet May Slow Development, 2018). The study highlights how simple lifestyle changes, such as those suggested on the Mediterranean diet, can help reduce the risk of Alzheimer's and other cognitive declines.

This indicates that diet can have an impact on the leading two signifiers of the development of Alzheimer's disease. Just as diet can impact other areas of your health, it can affect your brain health as well. Cholesterol, blood sugar, and blood vessel health can contribute to your risk of developing Alzheimer's disease. The most common sources of fuel for the brain are fresh fruits vegetables that supply it with vital vitamins and nutrients. When processed foods, refined grains, and added sugars are consumed too often, this impairs the brain's functionality as these foods release toxins into the body. These toxins then cause widespread inflammation and the brain begins to build up plaque which causes a malfunction to cognitive ability (Nutrition and Dementia, 2019).

The Western diet consists of a number of foods that increase the risk of Alzheimer's disease such as processed meat, refined grains like white bread and pasta, and added sugar. Foods that contain diacetyl, which is a chemical commonly used in the refinement process, increase beta-amyloid plaque build-up in the brain. Microwaveable popcorn, margarine, and butter are some of the most consumed foods that contain this harmful chemical. It is no wonder that Alzheimer's is becoming one of the leading causes of death among Americans.

The Mediterranean diet, on the other hand, includes a wide range of foods that have been proven to boost memory and slow down cognitive decline. Dark leafy vegetables, fresh berries, extra virgin olive oil, and fresh fish contain brain-boosting vitamins and minerals that can improve brain health. The Mediterranean diet can help you make the necessary diet and lifestyle changes that can greatly decrease your risk of Alzheimer's.

Reduces Risk of Parkinson's Disease

Parkinson's disease is a slowly progressing neurodegenerative disorder that affects the dopamine-producing neurons in the brain. Those with Parkinson's disease will suffer from:

- Tremors
- Muscle stiffness
- Balance troubles
- Difficulty walking
- Depression
- Sleep problems
- Cognitive disruptions

There is no cure for Parkinson's and medications and therapies suggested for this condition only helps individuals manage symptoms, not slow or stop the progress of the disease. Genetics and environmental factors have been researched to better understand what causes one to develop Parkinson's disease. While genetics plays a factor in exposure to pesticides, herbicides, high cholesterol, low vitamin D levels, and limited physical activity can all increase the risk of Parkinson's disease.

Parkinson disease is also common among individuals who have a higher level of oxidative stress. This damages the cell is the brain and can result in serious cognitive and physical decline. Antioxidants can help reduce the risk of developing Parkinson's disease and can help repair damaged cells and form stronger connections in the brain.

The Mediterranean diet encourages the consumption of antioxidant-rich foods such as fresh fruits and vegetables. Eating organic and locally grown fruits and vegetables reduces the risk of toxin exposure from pesticides and herbicides.

Those with Parkinson's are often encouraged to change their diet so that it includes more healthy fats, like extra virgin olive oil, seeds, and nuts, fresh fruits, organic vegetables, and whole grains. This diet recommendation is the basis of the Mediterranean diet. Individuals are also encouraged to reduce the consumption of salt, sugar, and empty calorie foods. Which is also what the Mediterranean diet encourages.

Protects Against Type 2 Diabetes

The Mediterranean diet is the most recommended diet from health professionals for those diagnosed with Type 2 diabetes or prediabetes. The combination of healthy foods and regular exercise that the Mediterranean diet promotes are two of the key components to help individuals manage and even see a remission of symptoms.

Type 2 diabetes develops when your body is no longer able to produce or use the insulin produced properly. This causes blood sugar levels to spike to dangerous levels. Your blood sugar or glucose is what gives your body energy. It supplies fuel to your muscles, tissues, and cells so they are able to function properly. When glucose is released into the bloodstream it signals the pancreas to begin to produce insulin so that the cells in the body can properly absorb the glucose. When you have type 2 diabetes your pancreas is either not making enough insulin, and therefore your cells are not able to absorb enough of it, or the insulin is not being used properly so glucose is remaining in the body. A build-up of glucose in your body can cause a long list of health complications. The body may turn to use its own muscle and fat to get the energy it needs. Blood vessels can also become damaged which increases the risk of heart attack and stroke.

Those who are at the greatest risk of developing Type 2 diabetes include:

- Individuals who are overweight or obese
- Individuals who have limited physical activity.
- Individuals who have a family history of Type 2 diabetes
- Individuals who have insulin resistance

The most common symptoms of Type 2 diabetes include

- Excessive fatigue
- Frequent numbness of the hands or feet
- Tingling feelings in the hands and feet
- Regular headaches
- Vision difficulties
- Increase in urination
- Unquenchable thirst

Type 2 diabetes can go undetected for years. Many individuals are unaware of their condition until a serious health complication arises because of the condition. Those with Type 2 diabetes are at a greater risk of heart attack, stroke, organ damage, loss of vision, hearing loss, and many other health conditions that can decrease quality of life and shorten your life-span.

What you eat contributes to the production of insulin and how efficiently your body is able to utilize the insulin produced. Carbohydrates specifically are converted to glucose for the body to use as energy. Many individuals are eating too many unhealthy carbs causing the body to be thrown out of balance and blood sugar levels to rise and remain at an elevated level. The most common foods known to spike glucose levels are white bread, pasta, and sugary beverages. The excessive sugar and simple carbs found in these items cause the body to have a sudden increase in glucose which the body often cannot handle fast enough.

Carbohydrates themselves are not all bad and when you choose the right ones, they can help slow down the release of glucose making it easier for the body to absorb the energy. Complex carbs, which are found naturally in many fruits, vegetables, and whole grains, get slowly released into the bloodstream. Eating foods high in fiber also helps slow down the release of glucose.

Type 2 diabetes has been strongly connected with diet. Diets that are high in trans fat, sugar, simple carbohydrates, and sodium increase the risk of developing diabetes. Individuals who transition to a Mediterranean diet lowers their risk of Type 2 diabetes. Those who have been diagnosed with pre-diabetes, which is often a red flag diagnosis that almost always leads to a diagnosis of Type 2 diabetes, can reverse the diagnosis. Those who suffer from diabetes will often find that the Mediterranean diet can help them significantly reduce symptoms and take control of their insulin and blood sugar levels.

The Mediterranean diet encourages improvement in both diet and physical activity. These two components are the most important factors that will help you manage diabetic symptoms and reduce your risk of developing the condition.

Additional Benefits

Aside from the significant benefits to your heart and brain, the Mediterranean diet can significantly improve a number of other key factors in your life. Since the Mediterranean diet focuses on eating healthy, exercising, and connecting with others, you can see improvements to your mental health, physical health, and will often feel like you're living a more satisfying life. Some of the other additional benefits you can experience when you transition to a Mediterranean diet are discussed below.

Longevity

The Mediterranean diet helps reduce the risk of many health issues. It's benefits to heart health, brain health, and mood all result in longer and more enjoyable life. When you eliminate the risk of developing certain conditions like cardiovascular disease, diabetes, and dementia you increase your life-span. But, eliminating these health risks is not the only cause for an increase in longevity on the Mediterranean diet. The increase in physical activity and deep social connection also plays a significant role in living a longer life.

Energy

Sticking to a Mediterranean diet focuses on fueling your body. Other diets focus on just filling your body and these are often done through empty calories. When your body is receiving the nutrients it needs, it can function properly and this results in you feeling more energized throughout the day. You won't need to rely on sugary drinks, excess caffeine, or sugar-filled energy bars to get you going and keep you going. You will feel less weighed down after you eat and this results in you being able to perform at increased levels of production.

Clear skin

Healthy skin begins from the inside out. When you are providing your body with wholesome foods this will radiate through your skin. The antioxidants in extra virgin olive oil alone are enough to keep your skin looking young and healthy. But, the Mediterranean diet includes a number of fresh fruits and vegetables that are packed with antioxidants. These antioxidants help repair damaged cells in the body and promote healthy cell growth. Eating a variety of healthy fats also keeps the skin elastic and can protect it from premature aging.

Better sleep

Sugar and caffeine can cause significant sleep disturbances. Additionally, other foods such as processed foods can make it more difficult for you to get the appropriate amount of sleep. When you are eating the right foods you can see a shift in your sleep patterns. Your body will want to rest to recover and properly absorb the vitamins and minerals consumed throughout the day. Your brain will be able to shift into sleep mode with ease because it has received the vitamins it needs to be able to function properly. When you get the right amount of sleep you will, in turn, have more energy the next day and this can also significantly improve your mood. The Mediterranean diet increases the consumption of nutrient-dense foods and avoids excess sugar and processed foods, which are known to cause sleep issues.

Additionally, the Mediterranean diet allows you to maintain a healthy weight which reduces your risk of developing sleep disorders like sleep apnea. Sleep apnea is common in individuals who are overweight and obese. It causes the airways to become blocked making it difficult to breathe. This results in you not taking in enough oxygen when you sleep which can cause you to wake up suddenly and frequently throughout the night.

Protects against cancer

Many plant-based foods, especially those in the yellow and orange color groups contain cancer-fighting agents. The increase of antioxidants consumed by eating fresh fruits and vegetables as well as whole grains can help protect the cells of the body from developing into cancer-causing cells. Drinking a glass of red wine also provides you with cancer-protecting compounds.

Maintain a healthy weight

On the Mediterranean diet, you will consume mostly whole, fresh foods. Eating more foods that are rich in vitamins, minerals, and nutrients is essential for maintaining a healthy weight. The diet is easy to adhere to and there are no calorie restrictions you need to strictly follow. This makes it a highly sustainable plan for those wanting to lose weight or maintaining a healthy weight. Keep in mind, this is not a loose weight fast option. This is a lifestyle diet that will allow you to maintain optimal health for years, not just a few months.

Chapter 7:
How to Make the Change

When you decide to make the change from an unhealthy or less desirable diet to the Mediterranean diet it is likely that you will notice positive changes in your health, mood, and energy, within the first 30 days. Making the transition to the Mediterranean diet doesn't have to mean changing everything all at once. Even starting out with just one small improvement can have significant effects. In this chapter, you will learn the steps you can take to begin to adopt a Mediterranean lifestyle. Making one small adjustment a week will provide you with an array of benefits that you may not notice immediately but will pay attention to as more time passes. In the next 30 days, you can see huge changes in your energy, sleep, and mood. When you are eating the right foods, everything else with your health and well being seems to adjust accordingly.

Breakfast is Essential

Eating a hearty breakfast that consists of whole grains, fruits, and fiber-rich foods is how many Mediterraneans start their day. Eating a healthy and filling breakfast will fuel you for the first half of your day and keep you full until lunch. Many people are so accustomed to rushing out the door that they skip breakfast or default to grabbing a sugary pastry while they are out and about. The problem with these breakfast pastries is they are often loaded with empty calories. They may provide you with a quick jolt of energy but will often lead to a crash shortly after.

When you eat a breakfast that is full of wholesome foods, you set the standard for how you will eat the rest of the day. Those who tend to skip breakfast are more likely to snack on unhealthy foods throughout the morning and then by lunch choose something quick and convenient instead of healthy and filling. Make it a priority to eat a breakfast that will provide you with enough fuel for the morning. High fiber foods will keep you feeling full for longer so you can avoid reaching for something to snack on before lunch.

Tips for Making Breakfast a Habit

- Eat a little from each major group: fresh fruits, vegetables, healthy fats, whole grains, and a small bit of protein like an egg.

- Make breakfast the simplest meal of the day. During the workweek you want breakfast to be a healthy and quick decision. On the weekend, plan for more elaborate breakfast or brunches that you can enjoy with your family.

- Use leftover whole grains to create savory oatmeal inspired dish or season with cinnamon and top with fresh berries.

Eat Plenty of Vegetables

There is really no restriction on the number of vegetables you can eat with the Mediterranean diet. What matters is that you are eating a wide variety of vegetables and choosing from different colored groups. Vegetables will provide you with most of the nutrients and vitamins your body needs to stay healthy.

Tips to add more vegetables to your meals:

- You can eat a number of raw vegetables as a snack throughout the day. Even a plate of fresh sliced tomatoes with crumbled feta cheese or sliced mozzarella and drizzle with olive oil and balsamic vinegar is a simple and delicious snack idea.

- Replace your go-to meat toppings for veggies. If you are used to eating pizza with sausage, pepperoni or bacon (or all three), change it up and pile on the mushrooms, peppers, onions, and spinach instead!

- Eat your vegetables first. Start your meals with a salad and then eat any side of vegetables before you cut into your steak, chicken, or consume your pasta. When you eat your vegetables first you will ensure that you are eating them all and you will find that you get full enough and are satisfied with just those.

- Dedicate one day a week for vegetarian meals. Make it a habit to create meals that are built around beans and legumes as your main source of protein. And don't scrimp on the vegetables when you do! If going vegetarian for a full day seems too challenging then start off with one meal a week that is strictly vegetarian, then add another, and another. Soon you will be so used to vegetarian meals that you will plan them without even thinking twice about it.

Include Seafood in Your Meals at Least Twice a Week

Most fish enjoyed on the Mediterranean diet are packed with beneficial Omega-3s, which are fatty acids that promote brain health. Regular consumption of fish can also help reduce inflammation in the body and keep your cholesterol levels in check. On the Mediterranean diet, fish is used to take the place of red meat and but is not consumed in large quantities. You want to include two to three servings of fish in your meal plan a week but, these should be small portions. Fish, like grains and red meat, are often more of a side to compliment the vegetables. Choose fish like salmon, tuna, mackerel, and sardines as your source of lean protein and consider other seafood items like shrimp, scallops, and mussels for your meals.

Tips for adding seafood to your meals:

- Choose wild-caught fish or buy directly from the fish market. This will keep the price low and ensure that your fish was caught that day.

- Don't limit yourself to just fish. Mediterraneans enjoy shrimp, oysters, mussels, and octopus regularly.

- Fish can be easily used in place of many recipes that call for chicken or red meat.

- Fish tend to not need a great deal of flavoring. Most of the time it can be served with a drizzle of olive oil and lemon juice.

Enjoy Dairy Moderately

Dairy provides you with plenty of calcium which your body needs to maintain optimal functionality. But, unlike how Western diets incorporate large quantities of dairy daily, the

Mediterranean diet encourages moderate consumption of dairy products. Note, dairy included in the Mediterranean diet is often a variety of cheeses that are served on top of salads. Yogurt is also enjoyed regularly and provides you with additional probiotics. Dairy products should be low-fat or nonfat. You don't need the extra fat from your dairy as you will eat more nuts, seeds, and olive oil which will provide you with enough of the healthy fats.

Tips to enjoy dairy in moderation:

- Add dairy on top of salads instead of in pasta dishes.

- Many kinds of cheese pair well with sweet fruits like grapes and strawberries.

- Enjoy yogurt for breakfast or dessert with fresh berries.

- Limit drinking milk on a daily basis. When you do choose milk go for the low-fat or nonfat options. Or simply swap out your typical cow's milk for organic soy milk.

Enjoy Dessert

The Mediterranean diet is all about enjoying your food so dessert is often served after dinners, especially when there's company. Desserts, however, are not cakes or baked goods. Most desserts served after dinner consist of fresh fruit and nuts.

Other pastries are enjoyed most of which are made with thin pieces of dough, or phyllo dough, and are stuffed with nuts like pistachios and walnuts, honey, and fruits. They are also prepared and cut into bite-sized pieces. It is not likely that even when serving up a dessert like these that you will need a fork to eat it with. Keeping the serving size small eliminates going overboard with the dessert.

Tips for dessert on the Mediterranean diet:

- Serve fresh sliced fruits like strawberries, apples, figs, and grapes after your meals.

- Make fruit-filled pies with a whole grain crust.

- Tart cherries served with greek yogurt and drizzle of honey is the perfect way to end a delightful dinner.

- Keep the desert portion small and allow for easy sharing.

- Make your own ice cream for dessert by blending up ripe bananas and folding in nuts or other slices of fruit. Then freeze for a few hours and enjoy.

Eat Healthy Fats

If you were to ask individuals of the Mediterranean how much olive oil they consume a day you might be surprised. Many consume up to a full cup of oil a day and others even more. This isn't something you would want to do with refined oils but with high-quality, unrefined oil, you can consume more without fear of negative effects. The price for extra olive oil might be out of your budget to use it as a cooking oil. Extra virgin olive oil should be reserved for drizzling on top of meals, dipping bread, and salad dressing. For cooking, go with a more affordable but still high-quality virgin olive oil. Virgin olive oil is still unrefined so it contains a high quantity of the healthy fatty acids and antioxidants in it but it has less of a flavor and aroma. Other healthy fats include nuts, seeds, and avocados. Almonds, macadamia nuts, and walnuts are included in many recipes from the Mediterranean region. They are also used for quick snack items to be enjoyed at any time of the day.

Tips for eating more of the right healthy fats:

- Top salads with extra virgin olive oil and balsamic vinegar or a dash of pepper.

- Use extra virgin olive oil in replace of condiments like ketchup. You can drizzle olive oil of steamed or raw vegetables, seafood, whole grains, and red meats.

- Use mashed avocado in recipes where you would typically use store-bought mayonnaise.

- Use virgin olive oil in place of butter or margarine when cooking.

Stock Up on Spices and Herbs

Salt is used minimally in Mediterranean recipes, and in most cases, it is left out completely. Instead, a combination of different herbs and spices is used in most recipes so the salt is neither needed or missed. Fresh herbs are ideal and can easily be ground up in your own kitchen when dried. Herbs provide you with additional minerals and nutrients that can boost your immunity and overall health.

You may find that some Mediterranean recipes have a long list of herbs and spices and others may only use one or two. This allows you to create a wide range of dishes, using many of the same base ingredients, but completely different flavor profiles.

Tips for using spices in your meals:

- Make batches of spice blends to have ready to use in the kitchen. Some simple spices blends to try:

    1. Taco seasoning - 1 Tablespoon chili

powder. ½ Teaspoon onion powder, garlic powder, dried oregano, and sea salt. ½ Tablespoon cumin. ¼ Teaspoon red pepper flake and cayenne pepper.

2. Chinese five spices - 1 Tablespoon ground cloves, cinnamon, ginger, and star anise seeds. 1 Teaspoon black pepper.

3. Italian season - 2 Tablespoons of dried basil, parsley, and oregano. 1 Tablespoon of dried rosemary, thyme, and chili flakes. 1 Teaspoon of garlic powder.

- Experiment with different spices. Cinnamon is a common household spice but it is not used in many savory dishes. Adding a little cinnamon to bar-b-que recipes or stews gives the meal a new and delightful flavor.

- Learn about spices from around the world. There are plenty of spices out there from turmeric to ginger that not only go well in a variety of dishes but also provide a substantial number of health benefits.

Grow Your Own

Even if you don't have a natural green thumb you can easily grow any number of your own fresh herbs and even a few vegetables to consume on the Mediterranean diet. Herbs like Oregano cilantro, basil, mint, and parsley can be kept on your kitchen counter and used when you need them. You can also easily create your own dried and ground herbs to store in your pantry. All you need is a mortar and pestle to ground herbs that you have hung and let dry.

If you have a yard, you can dedicate a small area for growing various fruits or vegetables. Tomatoes, cucumbers, peppers, squash, and spinach are great starters that you can grow on your own. Many major cities offer shared garden spaces that you can use to grow your own plants in if you don't have a space of your own.

Additionally, many areas in the United States have a Community Supported Agriculture program. These programs allow you to pay a fee and they will provide you with seasonal fresh fruits and vegetables throughout the year. The produce is usually grown from a local family farm. You can often find options for weekly, monthly or seasonal subscriptions. This is an ideal option for those who either don't have the space for gardening or who do not have an option for starting their own garden.

Chapter 8:
The Best Mediterranean Diet Breakfasts

Breakfast is a vital part of your day. When you skip breakfast you deprive your body of vital nutrients and minerals it needs. After a long night of rest, your body needs to be replenished and if you skip breakfast you're setting yourself up for fatigue and mood swings. On the Mediterranean diet, breakfast tends to be simple but nutritious. The recipes in this chapter will give a number of breakfast ideas that you can use any day of the week!

Caprese Poached Eggs

This breakfast dish is a twist on traditional Eggs Benedict. It replaces the Hollandaise sauce with a refreshing pesto sauce and substitutes in tomatoes instead of bacon or ham.

Serving Size: 2

Nutritional Information:

Calories - 357

Carbs - 19 g

Protein - 23 g

Fat - 21.5 g

Cook Time: 10 minutes

Ingredients:

- 1 tablespoon white vinegar (distilled)
- 4 eggs
- 1 tomato (sliced)
- 2 mozzarella cheese slices (1 ounce each)
- 4 teaspoon pesto
- 2 whole wheat English muffins
- 2 teaspoons sea salt

Directions:

1. Place a large saucepan on your stove and fill it with 3 inches of water. Turn the heat to high so that the water can come to a boil. Once the water is boiling add the tablespoon of vinegar to the saucepan and the salt, reduce the heat to medium-low so the water maintains a gentle boil.

2. As the water simmers, prepare your English muffins. Cut the muffins in half lengthwise. Place a slice of the mozzarella cheese on each muffin half then layer on a slice of tomato. Place the muffins on a cooking sheet and place them in your boiler. If you have a toaster oven you can use that instead of your broiler. Allow the muffins to toast up and the cheese to soften. This should take about 5 minutes.

3. As the muffins toast, crack an egg into a small bowl. Hold the bowl over the saucepan with the simmering water. Slowly pour the egg into the water, being careful not to break the yolk. Then repeat with the other three eggs. Once all eggs are in the water allow them to poach for about 3 minutes. The egg whites should be firm and fluffy.

4. As the eggs cook, place a few paper towels on a plate. Use a slotted spoon to transfer your cooked eggs to the plate to remove any excess water.

5. Remove your English muffin from the boiler or toaster oven.

6. Carefully transfer the muffin halves to a serving plate and place a poached egg on each half.

7. Take your pesto sauce and top each muffin with a tablespoon of the sauce. Serve and enjoy!

Sautéed Greens and Eggs

The filling leafy greens and eggs dish comes together in less than 20 minutes. You can store leftovers in your refrigerator for up to four days in an airtight container.

Serving Size: 4

Nutritional Information:

Calories - 152

Carbs - 3 g

Protein - 9.2 g

Fat - 11.9 g

Cook Time: 15 minutes

Ingredients:

- 1 tablespoon virgin olive oil
- 4 eggs
- 2 cups rainbow chard
- 1 cup spinach
- ½ cup arugula
- 2 garlic cloves (minced)
- ½ cup feta cheese
- ½ teaspoon sea salt
- ½ teaspoon black pepper

Directions:

1. Place a large skillet on your stove with the tablespoon of virgin olive oil. Turn the heat on to medium-high.

2. As the skillet is heating, break your eggs into a medium-sized mixing bowl and use a fork to beat the eggs. Set to the side.

3. Your skillet should be nice and hot now. Add in your rainbow chard, spinach, and arugula and allow the greens to sauté for about 5 minutes. Once the greens are nice and tender, add your minced garlic to the skillet and cook for two minutes.

4. Take your egg mixture and pour it into the skillet with your greens. Then sprinkle your feta cheese over top.

5. Cover the skillet with a lid and allow to cook for 6 minutes.

6. Once the eggs have cooked thoroughly, uncover the skillet and sprinkle the sea salt and black pepper over top.

7. Divide the mixture into four equal portions and serve!

Breakfast Pizza

This healthy version of breakfast pizza uses whole-wheat pita and is loaded with vegetables. This is an easy make and go recipe but is much better enjoyed on a morning where you can sit and share with the rest of the family. You can also add on some tuna or shrimp for a great lunch option!

Serving Size: 4

Nutritional Information:

Calories - 361

Carbs - 24.3 g

Protein - 12 g

Fat - 26 g

Cook Time: 20 minutes

Ingredients:

- 2 tablespoons virgin olive oil
- 4 eggs
- ¼ onion (chopped)
- ½ tomato (diced)
- ½ cup spinach (chopped)
- ½ cup mushroom (chopped)
- 1 avocado (pit and peel removed, sliced)

- 2 tablespoons pesto

- 2 pita bread

- ½ cup mozzarella cheese (shredded)

Directions:

1. Begin by lining a cookie sheet with parchment paper and set it to the side.

2. Start getting your oven nice and hot by preheating it to 350 degrees F.

3. Take a large skillet and place it on top of your stove. Pour in 1 tablespoon of the virgin olive oil. Turn the heat to medium-high. Add the chopped onions to your skillet and let them cook for 5 minutes. The onions should be translucent. Transfer the onions to a small bowl and set to the side.

4. Add the remaining 1 tablespoon of olive oil to the skillet.

5. In a mixing bowl crack the eggs and beat together with a fork. Pour the mixture into the skillet. Let the eggs cook for about 5 minutes, stir occasionally so that they cook evenly. Turn off the heat when they are cooked completely.

6. Take your prepared cookie sheet and place the pita bread on it. Spread a tablespoon of

your pesto on each pita. Top each pita with half the spinach, eggs, onions, tomatoes, mushrooms, and mozzarella cheese.

7. Place the cookie sheet into the oven for 10 minutes.

8. Remove the cookie sheet from the oven, then lay the sliced avocado over the top and enjoy!

Caprese on Sourdough

Sourdough is often served with most meals in Mediterranean countries. This super simple recipe uses it as one of the main ingredients but sticks to its traditional usage by topping it with olive oil, tomato, and mozzarella.

Serving Size: 4

Nutritional Information:

Calories - 196

Carbs - 17.2 g

Protein - 11.3 g

Fat - 9 g

Cook Time: 10 minutes

Ingredients:

- 1 tablespoon extra-virgin olive oil
- 1 garlic clove (peeled)
- 1 tomato (sliced)
- 4 thick slices of mozzarella cheese
- 8 basil leaves (fresh)
- 1 teaspoon oregano
- 1 tablespoon balsamic vinegar
- 4 slices of sourdough bread

Directions:

1. Begin by toasting your sourdough bread. This is easiest to do if you have a toaster oven, but you can also place them on a baking sheet and place them under your broiler for a minute or two, flip them so that each side is toasted.

2. Once your sourdough is nicely toasted take your peeled garlic clove and rub one side of each slice of bread.

3. Place two basil leaves on each piece of sourdough and a slice or two of tomatoes. Top with a thick slice of mozzarella cheese.

4. Drizzle a little bit of the olive oil and balsamic vinegar over top. Finish each slice with a sprinkle of oregano.

Mediterranean Inspired Breakfast Quinoa

This is a great alternative to your traditional oatmeal recipes. You can easily change this recipe up and add in some raisins or apricots instead of the apples or in addition to!

Serving Size: 4

Nutritional Information:

Calories - 225

Carbs - 37.2 g

Protein - 8.1 g

Fat - 5.3 g

Cook Time: 35 minutes

Ingredients:

- 1 cup quinoa (cooked)
- 2 cups low-fat milk
- 3 Medjool dates (pitted, chopped fine)
- 1 apple (cored, chopped)
- ¼ cup almonds (chopped)
- 1 teaspoon pure vanilla extract
- 1 teaspoon cinnamon (ground)
- 2 tablespoon honey (optional)

Directions:

1. Place a medium-sized skillet on your stove. Add in your chopped almonds, turn the heat to medium, and allow them to toast for about 5 minutes. When they are a nice golden brown turn the heat off and set them to the side.

2. Next, take a medium-sized saucepan and place it on your stove. Turn up the heat just a bit to medium-high. Add in your quinoa and cinnamon and warm for 3 minutes. Then pour in the milk and add your chopped apple. Wait for it to come to a boil. Once at a steady boil, cover the saucepan and reduce the heat to medium-low. Let all the flavors simmer for 20 minutes. Then add in the vanilla, dates, and half the toasted almost. Stir everything and cook for another 2 minutes.

3. Remove the from the heat and divide into four equal portions. Top with the remaining almonds and drizzle honey over top if you like it to be a little sweeter.

Eggs Florentine

Eggs Florentine is a light yet filling breakfast. It is packed with fresh spinach, mushroom, onions, and garlic and topped off with tomatoes and feta.

Serving Size: 4

Nutritional Information:

Calories - 174

Carbs - 6.1 g

Protein - 11.2 g

Fat - 12.3 g

Cook Time: 20 minutes

Ingredients:

- 1 tablespoon virgin olive oil
- 6 eggs
- 2 garlic cloves (minced)
- ½ onion (finely diced)
- ½ cup mushrooms (sliced)
- 2 cups spinach (chopped)
- 2 tomatoes (diced)
- 1 teaspoon oregano (dried)
- 1 teaspoon basil (dried)
- ¼ cup feta (crumbles)
- ¼ teaspoon black pepper

Directions:

1. Place a large skillet on your stove with the virgin olive oil in it. Turn the heat to medium. Add the garlic and diced onions to the skillet. Let the flavors of the onion and garlic cook together for 2 minutes then add the mushroom and spinach and cook for another 5 minutes.

2. As the spinach and mushrooms cook, crack your eggs into a small mixing bowl and lightly beat them with a fork. Once the spinach has wilted, pour the egg mixture into the skillet. Sprinkle on the oregano, basil, and black pepper. Cover the skillet and allow the eggs to cook for about 3 to 5 minutes, just until they are firm enough to flip.

3. Once you have flipped your eggs sprinkle the crumbled feta and tomatoes on top and cook for another 5 minutes.

4. Once everything has cooked thoroughly turn off the heat and cut into 4 equal portions and enjoy.

Shakshuka

This is a Mediterranean twist on a traditional North African dish. You will want to use an oven-safe skillet when you begin this recipe so you can easily transfer the meal to the oven to finish cooking. Feel free to add in additional veggies of your liking! This is a recipe that can be savored for breakfast, brunch, or dinner, and it serves up a lot so it is perfect to enjoy with company.

Serving Size: 6

Nutritional Information:

Calories - 169

Carbs - 13.2 g

Protein - 8.6 g

Fat - 10.3 g

Cook Time: 50 minutes

Ingredients:

- 2 tablespoons virgin olive oil
- 6 eggs
- 1 onion (diced)
- 2 garlic cloves (minced)
- ½ cup mushrooms (sliced)
- 1 yellow bell pepper (diced)

- 1 red bell pepper (diced)
- 1 green bell pepper (diced)
- 1 cup spinach (chopped)
- 3 ½ cups plum tomatoes (diced)
- ¼ teaspoon cayenne pepper
- ¼ teaspoon cinnamon (ground)
- 1 teaspoon cumin
- ½ teaspoon paprika
- ½ teaspoon turmeric (ground)
- ½ teaspoon black pepper
- 2 tablespoons feta (crumbled)
- ½ cup water (or as needed)

Directions:

1. Place an oven-safe skillet on the stove, a cast-iron skillet is ideal for this dish. Add in the virgin olive oil and turn the heat all the way to medium-high, allow the oil to heat for about 2 minutes. Add in the diced onions, minced garlic, and sliced mushrooms and cook for about 10 minutes. You want the onions to begin to caramelize and the mushroom to release their liquids.

2. Add the red, yellow, and green bell peppers, and spinach to the skillet.

Sprinkle on the cayenne pepper, cinnamon, cumin, paprika, turmeric, and black pepper. Stir everything together and cook for another 5 minutes.

3. Pour in a half cup of water to the skillet and then add the diced tomatoes. Bring the water to a gentle simmer. Reduce the heat to medium, and allow everything to simmer for 15 minutes. Stir occasionally, if the mixture begins to thicken too much add a little more water.

4. As you let the vegetables simmer preheat your oven to 375 degrees F.

5. Create six wells into the vegetable mixture and carefully crack one egg into each well. You can first crack your eggs into a small dish and then gently slide them into the wells to ensure you do not break the yolks as place your eggs.

6. Once you have cracked all the eggs transfer your skillet into the oven. Bake long enough for the eggs to cook to your preference. For a slightly runny yolk, this should be about 10 minutes.

7. Remove the skillet from the oven and divide into six equal portions. Each portion should have an egg. Top with crumbled feta and enjoy!

Egg White Breakfast Sandwich

This is a quick and easy breakfast sandwich that you can make any day of the week.

Serving Size: 2

Nutritional Information:

Calories - 261

Carbs - 31.8 g

Protein - 14.6 g

Fat - 9.2 g

Cook Time: 10 minutes

Ingredients:

- 1 tablespoon virgin olive oil
- 4 egg whites
- ½ cup spinach
- 1 tomato (sliced)
- 2 whole-grain English muffins

Directions:

1. Place a medium-sized skillet on your stove and turn the heat to medium. Pour in the virgin olive oil to warm.

2. Lightly beat your egg whites in a small mixing bowl and then pour into your skillet. Allow the egg whites to cook for

108

about 3 minutes, flip and cook for 3 more minutes on the other side. When fully cooked, the whites should be firm and fluffy. Turn off the heat.

3. Slice your English muffins in half and place them in your toaster oven. Remove once toasted.

4. Divide your cooked egg whites into two equal portions and place on one slice of your toasted English muffin. Layer on your sliced tomatoes and spinach. Place the other half of your English muffin on top and enjoy!

Mediterranean Egg Wrap

Sun-dried tomatoes are common in a number of Mediterranean recipes. They offer a wide range of antioxidants that help fight free radicals. This recipe pairs sun-dried tomatoes with feta and spinach for a healthy and flavorful breakfast. You can easily make this for one by cutting the recipe in half.

Serving Size: 2

Nutritional Information:

Calories - 371

Carbs - 19.9 g

Protein - 20 g

Fat - 24.8 g

Cook Time: 10 minutes

Ingredients:

- 1 tablespoon virgin olive oil
- 4 eggs
- 2 cups spinach (chopped)
- 2 sundried tomatoes (chopped)
- 2 tomatoes (diced)
- ½ cup feta cheese (crumbled)
- 2 whole-wheat tortillas

Directions:

1. Begin by placing a large skillet on your stove. Pour in the virgin olive oil and turn up the heat to medium-high. While waiting for the oil to heat up, crack your eggs in a small mixing bowl and use a fork to lightly beat the eggs together. Set the eggs to the side.

2. Once the oil in the skillet has been heating up for a few minutes add in your spinach and sundried tomatoes. Allow the spinach to cook for about 3 minutes or until it begins to wilt. Then pour in the eggs. Use a spatula to scramble the mixture as it cooks. Let the eggs cook for about 3 minutes. Sprinkle on the feta cheese and cook for another minute. Turn the heat all the way off.

3. Warm your tortillas for about 30 seconds in your microwave. Then divide your egg mixture between the two tortillas. Top each with diced tomatoes.

4. Fold in two sides of your tortilla and then roll like a burrito.

5. You can place it in a warm skillet so that the wrap holds its shape better or you can simply enjoy it as is!

Fruits, Oats, and Yogurt Parfait

This is a delightful and refreshing light breakfast. You can modify it to your preference and add a variety of fruits. What is great about this healthy breakfast is that it can also be enjoyed as a dessert or snack.

Serving Size: 1

Nutritional Information:

Calories - 376

Carbs - 38.8 g

Protein - 19.4 g

Fat - 18.3 g

Cook Time: 15 minutes

Ingredients:

- ½ cup whole-grain oats
- ¼ cup walnuts (chopped)
- 1 teaspoon honey
- 1 cup strawberries (fresh, sliced)
- ½ cup low-fat Greek yogurt

Directions:

1. Begin by getting your oven nice and hot. Preheat it to 325 degrees F.

2. Take a non-stick baking sheet and spread your whole grain oats and chopped walnuts across the sheet. Place the baking sheet into your oven and toast the oats and walnuts for 10 minutes. Once they have toasted to a nice crisp texture, remove from the oven and set to the side to cool.

3. Take a small microwaveable bowl and add in your teaspoon of honey. Heat the honey for 30 seconds. Remove from the microwave and add in your sliced strawberries. Stir the strawberries carefully to coat each evenly.

4. Take a parfait dish and add a fourth of the strawberry and honey mixture to the bottom. Then add a tablespoon of the greek yogurt followed by a sprinkle of the oats and walnuts. Repeat this process so that all your ingredients are layered and used. Then grab a spoon and enjoy!

Chapter 9:
The Best Mediterranean Diet Lunch

Unlike the way most Westerners enjoy lunch, on the Mediterranean diet lunch is a time to pause and take a break from a long workday. Enjoy any of the recipes in this chapter for a healthy lunch that you will want to stop and savor. Many of the recipes here can also be used as snack options or dinner ideas. Feel free to modify them as you like and add in more vegetables if you desire.

Italian Bean Soup

This hearty and filling soup makes for a great lunch or even dinner option. You can also add in a number of other vegetables for more nutrients such as carrots, bell peppers, potatoes, or zucchini.

Serving Size: 4

Nutritional Information:

Calories - 164

Carbs - 25.6 g

Protein - 8.1 g

Fat - 3.8 g

Cook Time: 15 minutes

Ingredients:

- 1 tablespoon virgin olive oil
- 1 onion (diced)
- 2 garlic cloves (minced)
- 2 cups tomato sauce (homemade or 1 can of low-sodium organic canned tomato sauce)
- 3 cups cooked cannellini beans (or about 24 ounces of canned beans that have been drained and rinsed)
- 1 tablespoon basil (dried)

- ½ teaspoon oregano
- ¼ teaspoon black pepper

Directions:

1. Take a large soup or stockpot and place it on your stove. Turn the heat all the way up to medium-high and pour in the virgin olive oil. Allow the oil to heat slightly before adding your diced onions to the pot. Sautee for 3 minutes and then add the garlic. Let the flavors come together for 2 minutes.

2. Add the cannellini beans, basil, oregano, and black pepper to the pot. Stir everything together then pour over the tomato sauce. Allow the sauce to come to a steady simmer. Reduce the heat to medium-low. Cover your pot so the flavors can simmer together for 5 minutes.

3. Uncover the pot and allow the aroma to fill your kitchen. Then, take a ladle and fill your soup bowls! Grab a soup spoon and enjoy!

Traditional Hummus

Hummus is a popular dish in the Mediterranean. This simple recipe yields a lot so you can easily use it for lunch served with raw veggies and warm pita. You can also use it to top wraps, sandwiches, and more. The recipes call for chickpeas, also known as garbanzo beans, so look for both names when shopping. You can use canned beans or dry cooked beans.

Serving Size: 20 (2 tablespoons per serving)

Nutritional Information:

Calories - 113

Carbs - 15.6 g

Protein - 5.1 g

Fat - 3.7 g

Cook Time: 5 minutes

Ingredients:

- 2 tablespoons extra virgin olive oil
- 2 ½ cups chickpeas (cooked)
- 2 garlic cloves
- 4 tablespoons lemon juice (fresh)
- 2 tablespoons tahini
- ¼ teaspoon black pepper

Directions:

1. Combine the chickpeas, garlic, lemon juice, tahini, and black pepper into your blender. Blend on high until you have a smooth and creamy mixture. If the mixture is too thick for your liking, add a tablespoon of water as needed.

2. Transfer the hummus to an airtight container and store it in your refrigerator until ready to serve.

3. You can store the hummus for up to seven days.

4. Serve with raw vegetables like carrots, bell pepper, and cucumbers, or whole-grain crackers or warm pita bread.

Chicken Quinoa Salad

This Mediterranean style quinoa salad is great for lunch but, you can leave out the chicken and use it as a healthy side dish for dinner as well. Don't let the long list of ingredients scare you, most are a variety of spices and herbs that give this dish a flavorful punch!

Serving Size: 8

Nutritional Information:

Calories - 243

Carbs - 19.1 g

Protein - 17.2 g

Fat - 11.2 g

Cook Time: 60 minutes

Ingredients:

- 2 tablespoons virgin olive oil
- 2 tablespoons extra virgin olive oil
- 2 chicken breasts (skinless, boneless)
- 1 red onion (diced)
- 1 garlic clove (minced)
- 1 green bell pepper (diced)
- ½ cup Kalamata olives (chopped)
- ⅔ cup lemon juice (fresh squeezed)

- 1 tablespoon balsamic vinegar
- 1 cup quinoa
- ¼ cup feta cheese (crumbled)
- 1 teaspoon sage (dried)
- 1 teaspoon garlic powder
- 1 teaspoon thyme (dried)
- 1 teaspoon parsley (dried)
- 1 teaspoon basil (dried)
- ½ teaspoon marjoram (dried)
- 1 teaspoon rosemary (dried)
- 1 teaspoon paprika (dried)
- ½ teaspoon ginger (dried)
- 1 teaspoon dried onion
- ½ teaspoon celery salt
- 1 teaspoon sea salt
- 1 teaspoon black pepper
- 2 cups water

Directions:

1. Pour the 2 cups of water in a medium pot and place it on your stove. Turn up the heat all the way to medium-high and add in the dried sage, garlic powder, thyme, parsley, basil, marjoram, rosemary,

paprika, ginger, onion, celery salt, sea salt, and black pepper. Bring to a boil.

2. Add your quinoa in the pot, allow the water to come back up to a boil before you reduce the heat to medium-low. Cover and allow the quinoa to simmer for 25 minutes so it can cook and absorb all the flavors from the spices and herbs.

3. As the quinoa cooks, place a large skillet on your stove and add in 2 tablespoons of your virgin olive oil. Turn the heat to medium. Place your boneless, skinless chicken breast to the skillet and cook for 10 minutes on each side. The internal temperature of your chicken should reach 165 degrees F.

4. When chicken is cooked to the appropriate temperature, remove them from the skillet. Let the chicken cool enough for you to handle, then cut them into bite-size cubes and transfer to a large mixing bowl.

5. When quinoa has absorbed all the water, add this to the mixing bowl with the chicken.

6. Add your diced onions, green bell pepper, olives, and feta cheese into the large mixing bowl. Toss everything together.

7. Drizzle the 2 tablespoons of extra virgin olive oil, freshly squeezed lemon juice, and balsamic vinegar over top. Give the mixture another stir and enjoy.

8. Store leftovers in your refrigerator for up to five days. You can enjoy this reheated or cold.

Greek Inspired Potatoes

This Greek-inspired potato recipe makes a great lunch option but can also be served as a side to your main course dinner. These pair well with fresh fish like salmon or turbot. You can also add in some extra vegetables like carrots, zucchini, or cauliflower.

Serving Size: 4

Nutritional Information:

Calories - 340

Carbs - 52.1 g

Protein - 5.7 g

Fat - 13.2 g

Cook Time: 2 hours

Ingredients:

- ¼ cup virgin olive oil

- 2 garlic cloves (minced)

- 6 potatoes (peeled, cut into large cubes or quartered)

- ¼ cup lemon Juice (fresh squeezed)

- 1 teaspoon thyme (dried)

- 1 teaspoon rosemary (dried)

- 1 tablespoon oregano

- ½ teaspoon sea salt
- ¼ teaspoon black pepper
- 1 ½ cups water

Directions:

1. You want to begin by preheating your oven to 350 degrees F.

2. While your oven is getting nice and hot, take a small mixing bowl and whisk together the olive oil, minced garlic, freshly squeezed lemon juice, dried thyme, rosemary, oregano, sea salt, black pepper, and water. Set to the side.

3. Place your cubed potatoes into a large mixing bowl and pour half of your olive oil and herb mixture into the bowl. Mix everything together so that the potatoes are nicely coated with the mixture.

4. Transfer the potatoes to a large baking dish, then pour over the remainder of the olive oil mixture. Cover the baking dish with foil and place it into your preheated oven. Bake for 1 ½ hours and stir occasionally. The potatoes should have a little bit of firmness to them when they are just about done. After they have cooked, covered for 1 ½ hours, uncover and bake for another 20 minutes.

5. Remove from your oven and enjoy. You can store leftover potatoes in an airtight container for up to five days in your refrigerator.

Lentil Soup

This Greek-inspired recipe is flavorful and filling. Brown lentils are a significant source of fiber and protein, which is necessary on the Mediterranean diet. Aside from the minerals and vitamins provided by lentils they also offer a nice earthy and rich flavor that makes for a great addition in soups and stews.

Serving Size: 4

Nutritional Information:

Calories - 128

Carbs - 13.2 g

Protein - 4.1 g

Fat - 7.2 g

Cook Time: 1 hour 20 minutes

Ingredients:

- 2 tablespoons virgin olive oil
- 1 cup brown lentils
- 2 garlic cloves (minced)
- 1 tablespoon tomato paste
- 1 red onion (minced)
- 1 carrot (chopped)
- 1 teaspoon oregano (dried)

- 1 teaspoon rosemary (dried)

- 2 bay leave

- ¼ teaspoon sea salt

- ¼ teaspoon black pepper

- 1 teaspoon balsamic vinegar (optional)

- 4 cups water

Directions:

1. Place the lentils into a medium-sized pot and fill with enough water so the lentils are covered a little over 1 inch. Turn the heat to medium-high and allow the water to come to a boil. Reduce the heat to medium so the lentils can cook for 10 minutes. Once the lentils are tender, drain the water and set to the side.

2. Pour the 2 tablespoons of virgin olive oil into a large saucepan on your stove. Turn the heat to medium and allow the oil to heat up for a few minutes. Add the minced garlic, red onions, and carrot to the pan. Allow them to cook for 5 minutes. The onions should be translucent.

3. Add the 4 cups of water to the saucepan along with the dried oregano, rosemary, and bay leaves. Allow the water to come to a boil then transfer the lentils to the

saucepan. Turn the heat down to medium-low, cover the saucepan, and allow everything to simmer for 10 minutes.

4. Uncover the pot and add in the tomato paste, sea salt, and black pepper. Place the lid back on the saucepan and cook for another 30 minutes. Stir occasionally, if the soup is becoming too thick then add in another cup of water.

5. Once the lentils have softened, turn off the heat and ladle into a bowl.

6. Top with a drizzle of balsamic vinegar if you desire and enjoy.

7. You can store leftovers in an airtight container in your refrigerator for up to five days.

White Bean Soup

Soups don't have to take all day to make. This easy and delicious soup recipe cooks up in about 35 minutes. While this recipe uses canned white kidney beans, you can use chickpeas or cannellini beans. You can also just as easily swap out the canned beans for about 4 cups of pre-soaked dried beans.

Serving Size: 4

Nutritional Information:

Calories - 185

Carbs - 23.8 g

Protein - 10.1 g

Fat - 5.2 g

Cook Time: 35 minutes

Ingredients:

- 1 tablespoon virgin olive oil
- 1 red onion (chopped)
- 1 garlic clove (minced)
- 1 celery stalk (chopped)
- 1 cup spinach (fresh, finely chopped)
- 1 tablespoon lemon juice (fresh squeezed)

- 2x 16-ounce cans white kidney beans (drained, rinsed)

- 2 cups chicken broth (or a 14-ounce can of low-sodium chicken broth)

- ¼ teaspoon thyme (dried)

- ½ teaspoon black pepper

- 1 ½ cups water

Directions:

1. Place a large saucepan on your stove. Add the virgin olive oil to your pan and turn the heat to medium-high. Add the celery, chopped onions, and minced garlic to the pan and allow them to cook for 5 minutes.

2. Add the white kidney beans, chicken broth, water, thyme, and black pepper to the saucepan. Allow the liquid to come to a boil, then reduce heat to medium-low and let the soup simmer for 15 minutes.

3. Transfer two cups of the bean and vegetables from the saucepan to a bowl. Use a slotted spoon to get as little of the liquid as possible. Set the bowl to the side.

4. Use an emulsion blender to blend the remaining soup mixture in the saucepan. You want to get a nice smooth consistency.

If you do not have an emulsion blender you can use a regular stand-alone blender. Just work in batches to blend everything. Once everything has been thoroughly blended, return back to your saucepan.

5. Add the 2 cups of beans and vegetable mixture that you removed earlier back into the soup. Bring the soup back up to a boil, stirring occasionally.

6. Add in the spinach to the soup; after 2 minutes it should begin to wilt.

7. Turn the heat all the way off, then stir in the lemon juice just before serving.

Whole Wheat Penne with Shrimp

This is a light pasta dish that can be modified to include more of your favorite vegetables. Broccoli, cauliflower, zucchini, and mushrooms are just a few delicious options to include. If you are not a big fan of shrimp, chicken breast or salmon can also work well in this recipe. What makes this dish so delicious is the simple red wine tomato sauce. It is bursting with flavor and you'll never miss that jarred pasta sauce one bit.

Serving Size: 4

Nutritional Information:

Calories - 331

Carbs - 14.7 g

Protein - 22.8 g

Fat - 8.9 g

Cook Time: 30 minutes

Ingredients:

- 2 tablespoon virgin olive oil
- 1 pound shrimp (peeled, deveined)
- ¼ red onion (chopped)
- 2 garlic cloves (chopped)
- 1 ½ cups tomatoes (diced)
- 1 cup parmesan cheese (gratedo

- 2 cups whole wheat penne pasta (16-ounce package)

- ¼ cup red wine

Directions:

1. Cook the whole wheat pasta according to package directions. For an even texture while, bring water to a full boil before adding the pasta, then reduce heat just enough so the water maintains a vigorous boil without spilling over the top of your pot. Pasta should cook in about 10 minutes. When pasta is cooked to your liking, drain the water, rinse with cold water, and set to the side.

2. Take a large skillet and place it on your stove with the 2 tablespoons of virgin olive oil in it. Turn the heat to medium and allow the oil to warn a little. You can do this step while you are waiting for your pasta to cook to save some time. Once the oil has heated for a minute or two add your chopped red onions and garlic to the pan. Cook for 5 minutes so the onions become tender.

3. Pour the red wine into the skillet and add your diced tomatoes. Allow everything to simmer for 10 minutes.

4. Add your shrimp to the skillet and mix everything together. Let the shrimp cook for about 5 minutes.

5. Add your pasta to the skillet. Stir and cook for 1 more minute. Turn the heat off.

6. Sprinkle your parmesan cheese over top and then divide into four equal portions.

Warm Cod Salad

This recipe is loaded with nutritious vegetables. It is a vibrant and filling meal perfect for lunch or dinner. Feel free to add in some jumbo shrimp or additional vegetables that you love! You can serve this dish as is or spoon on top of quinoa or whole grain rice.

Serving Size: 4

Nutritional Information:

Calories - 202

Carbs - 17.5 g

Protein - 23.8 g

Fat - 5.3 g

Cook Time: 25 minutes

Ingredients:

- 1 tablespoon virgin olive oil
- 4x 4-ounce cod fillets
- ¼ red onion (chopped fine)
- 2 garlic cloves (minced)
- ½ cup green olives (chopped)
- ½ cup cauliflower (florets chopped)
- 1 cup cherry tomatoes (halved)
- 1 carrot (diced)

- 1 zucchini (chopped)

- 1 red bell pepper (diced)

- 1 yellow bell pepper (diced)

- ½ cup broccoli (florets chopped)

- 1 celery stalk (chopped)

- 1 cup tomato sauce (low-sodium)

- ¼ cup balsamic vinegar

- 1 teaspoon oregano

- 1 teaspoon garlic powder

- 1 teaspoon paprika

- ½ teaspoon cayenne pepper

- ¼ teaspoon sea salt

- ¼ teaspoon black pepper

Directions:

1. Begin with a large skillet on your stove with the virgin olive oil in it. Turn the heat all the way up to medium-high, then add in the chopped onions and minced garlic. Cook the onions and garlic for about 5 minutes, stir frequently to avoid burning.

2. Once the onions are tender, pour in the tomato sauce, balsamic vinegar, and toss in the cherry tomatoes. Bring the sauce to a simmer, then add in cauliflower, carrots,

red and yellow bell peppers, zucchini, broccoli, and celery. Stir everything together, cover, and allow to simmer for 5 more minutes.

3. Add in the oregano, garlic powder, paprika, cayenne pepper, sea salt, and black pepper to the skillet. Stir everything again, then add the green olives. Place the cod fillets on top of the vegetables in the skillet. Reduce heat to medium, cover and cook for 5 minutes. Use a fork to flake apart the cod fillets. If they do not flake apart with ease, then allow them to cook for another 3 minutes.

4. Stir the cod into the rest of the veggies and then serve.

5. You can store any leftovers in an airtight container in your refrigerator for up to three days.

Mediterranean Barley Salad with Chicken

If you are looking for a lunch option that brings you plenty of flavors and balances your grain, proteins, and fresh vegetables portions, this is the ideal dish for you. This dish is meant to be served cold so you can easily store leftovers for lunch all week without worrying about reheating! You can also leave out the chicken and serve the barley as a delicious side dish for dinnertime.

Serving Size: 6

Nutritional Information:

Calories - 306

Carbs - 28.4

Protein - 22.4 g

Fat - 12.5 g

Cook Time: 45 minutes

Ingredients:

- 2 tablespoons extra virgin olive oil
- 2 tablespoons virgin olive oil
- 2 chicken breasts (boneless, skinless)
- 1 cup barley
- 6 sun-dried tomatoes (chopped)

- ½ cup black olives (chopped)

- 2 garlic cloves

- ½ cup cilantro (fresh, chopped fine)

- 1 tablespoon balsamic vinegar

- ½ teaspoon sea salt

- ½ teaspoon black pepper

- 2 ½ cups of water

Directions:

1. Place a pot that is medium-size on your stove and pour in the 2 ½ cups of water. You want to turn the heat all the way up to high, so the water comes to a boil quickly. When water is boiling, add the barley. Wait for the water to come back up to a boil before turning the heat down to medium-low. Place a lid on the pot and allow the barley to cook for 30 minutes. It should be slightly firm when done. Drain the water and transfer the barley to a large mixing bowl so it can cool.

2. As the barley is cooking or while cooling, heat a large skillet on your stove over medium heat. Add in 2 tablespoons of the virgin olive oil. Season your boneless, skinless chicken breast with sea salt and black pepper on each side. Then, place

your chicken breast into your heated skillet. Cover and cook for about 10 minutes on each side. The internal temperature should reach 165 degrees F.

3. Once the chicken is cooked to the appropriate temperature, remove it from the skillet so it can cool.

4. While waiting for the chicken to cool, you can make your sauce to go over the barley. Place the sun-dried tomatoes, garlic cloves, balsamic vinegar, and 2 tablespoons of the extra virgin olive oil in your blender or food processor. Puree the ingredients until you have a nice smooth mixture, then set to the side.

5. Once the chicken has cooled enough to handle dice the breast into small bite-size pieces. Add the chicken to the mixing bowl with the barley. Then pour your sauce mixture over top. Add in the chopped black olive and chopped cilantro. Use a large spoon to mix everything together. Cover the bowl with a lid or plastic wrap and store in your refrigerator until ready to serve.

Slow-Cooked Moroccan Chicken

This is a slow cooker recipe, so you will need a crockpot to bring this dish together. Slow cooking the chicken allows it to absorb all the flavors from the spices and herbs. Plus, it makes prepping lunch hassle-free since you can just combine all the ingredients and not have to touch it until it's done and ready to be portioned out.

Serving Size: 6

Nutritional Information:

Calories - 278

Carbs - 34.8 g

Protein - 26.3 g

Fat - 5.3 g

Cook Time: 6 hours 30 minutes

Ingredients:

- 2 chicken breasts (boneless, skinless, cut into 2-inch cubes)

- 15-ounce can garbanzo beans or chickpeas (drained, you can also use 2 cups of dried beans that have been pre-soaked overnight)

- 4 garlic cloves (chopped)

- 1 red onion (chopped)

- 2 cups tomatoes (diced)
- 3 peaches (peel and pit removed, sliced)
- 1 cup apricots (chopped)
- ⅓ cup almonds (slivers, toasted)
- ½ teaspoon cayenne pepper
- 1 teaspoon cinnamon (ground)
- ½ teaspoon coriander (ground)
- 2 teaspoon cumin (ground)
- 1 teaspoon ginger (ground)
- 1 tablespoon cornstarch
- 1 tablespoon warm water
- 2 cups chicken broth

Directions:

1. Add the cubed chicken breast, garlic, red onion, diced tomatoes, sliced peaches, garbanzos, chopped apricots, cayenne pepper, cinnamon, coriander, cumin, and ginger to your slow cooker. Pour the chicken broth over top. Place the lid on and set the temperature to low. Allow everything to cook for 6 hours.

2. After 6 hours, mix together the cornstarch and warm water in a small mixing bowl. Pour the cornstarch mixture into the slow

cooker and stir. Change the temperature to high and cook for another 30 minutes, or until the sauce has thickened.

3. Serve as is or spoon over quinoa or whole grain rice. Top with the toasted almonds just before serving.

Chapter 10:
The Best Mediterranean Diet Dinners

Dinner on the Mediterranean diet is a time that is shared with friends and family. These filling recipes focus on including a variety of vegetables and also offer different ways to include fish and beans into your meal plan. Remember to make dinner a special occasion every night of the week. Your meal should not just be good for your physical health but for your mental health as well. The recipes in this section can also be used for lunch ideas and a few can be used as breakfast or brunch!

Tilapia Florentine

Tilapia is a white flakey fish that is easy to find all year round. It is baked to perfection over a bed of spinach and seasoned vegetables. This light dinner option is the perfect meal to share and talk about your day with the rest of the family.

Serving Size: 4

Nutritional Information:

Calories - 174

Carbs - 3.9 g

Protein - 24.3 g

Fat - 7.6 g

Cook Time: 45 minutes

Ingredients:

- 1 tablespoon extra-virgin olive oil
- 4 tilapia fillets
- ¼ cup red onion (chopped)
- 1 garlic clove (minced)
- 1 ½ cups spinach (fresh)
- ¼ cup Kalamata olives (sliced)
- 1 lemon (¼ teaspoon grated lemon rind, freshly squeezed lemon juice)
- 2 tablespoon feta cheese (crumbled)
- ¼ teaspoon oregano (dried)

- ½ teaspoon paprika
- ½ teaspoon sea salt
- ¼ teaspoon black pepper

Directions:

1. You want to begin by first preheating your oven to 400 degrees F.

2. Next, place a large skillet on your stove and add in your tablespoon of olive oil. Turn the heat to medium. Add your chopped red onions and minced garlic to the skillet. Let them cook for about 5 minutes. Then add your spinach and cook for another 5 minutes.

3. Once the spinach has wilted add in the Kalamata olives, grated lemon rind, oregano, salt, black pepper, and crumbled feta cheese. Give everything a thorough stir and cook for another 5 minutes.

4. Take a baking dish, around 9x13 inches, and spread the spinach mixture evenly across the bottom. Place your tilapia fillets over the spinach. Squeeze the lemon juice over each fillet and sprinkle the paprika over top. Cover and place in your preheated oven. Allow the dish to bake for 20 minutes. Then uncover and bake for another 5 minutes.

Sheet Pan Chicken, Mediterranean Style

This dish is just as visually appealing as it is delightful to the taste buds. It offers a wide array of colors from the different vegetables and robust flavors from the herbs and spices. What is even better, sheet pan dinners make clean up a breeze so you can quickly be back spending time with your family and friends instead of doing mounds of dishes in the kitchen.

Serving Size: 4

Nutritional Information:

Calories - 427

Carbs - 35.1 g

Protein - 25.3 g

Fat - 23 g

Cook Time: 45 minutes

Ingredients:

- ¼ cup virgin olive oil
- 4 chicken thighs (skinless, boneless)
- 1 red onion (sliced)
- 1 pound small red potatoes (halved)
- 8 Kalamata olives (pitted, halved)

- 8 baby/mini bell peppers (seeds removed, cut lengthwise)

- 2 lemons (1 juiced, 1 sliced))

- 1 teaspoon oregano (dried)

- 1 teaspoon paprika

- 1 teaspoon tarragon (dried)

- ¼ cup feta cheese (crumbled)

- ½ teaspoon sea salt

- ½ teaspoon black pepper

- 2 tablespoon balsamic vinegar

Directions:

1. First, get your oven nice and hot by preheating it to 425 degrees F. Then line a baking sheet with foil. Be sure the baking sheet has a rim.

2. Combine the olive oil, freshly squeezed lemon juice, balsamic vinegar, oregano, paprika, tarragon, sea salt, and the black pepper in a large mixing bowl. Whisk everything together thoroughly. Then add in the onion slices, mini bell peppers, potatoes, and your boneless, skinless chicken thighs. Toss everything so it is all evenly coated with the olive oil.

3. Pour the vegetables and chicken thighs onto your foil-covered baking sheet. Lay the lemon slice on top. Place the baking sheet into your oven so everything can bake together nicely for 40 minutes.

4. Remove the baking sheet from the oven. You'll be tempted to try a little, but wait until you have topped it off with the Kalamata olives and crumbled feta cheese.

Lemon Caper Chicken

Serve this chicken dish with plenty of vegetables like broccoli, cauliflower or try the Greek inspired potatoes from the previous chapter. You can also serve this with a small serving of quinoa or whole grain rice and vegetables. This makes for an incredibly easy meal that can be served for dinner or lunch.

Serving Size: 4

Nutritional Information:

Calories - 182

Carbs - 3.4 g

Protein - 26.6 g

Fat - 8.2 g

Cook Time: 15 minutes

Ingredients:

- 2 tablespoon virgin olive oil
- 2 chicken breasts (boneless, skinless, cut in half, pound to ¾ an inch thick)
- ¼ cup capers
- 2 lemons (wedges)
- 1 teaspoon oregano
- 1 teaspoon basil
- ½ teaspoon black pepper

Directions:

1. Take a large skillet and place it on your stove and add the olive oil to it. Turn the heat to medium and allow it to warm up.

2. As the oil heats up season your chicken breast with the oregano, basil, and black pepper on each side.

3. Place your chicken breast into the hot skillet and cook on each side for five minutes.

4. Transfer the chicken from the skillet to your dinner plate. Top with capers and serve with a few lemon wedges.

Herb Roasted Chicken

Making a whole chicken allows you to have plenty for dinner and leftovers for lunch. You can easily store anything you don't eat at dinner in an airtight container or keep in your freezer for later use. This recipe uses fresh herbs and lemon to bring out irresistible flavors. It can be served alongside any vegetarian dish, shredded and used in salads or soups.

Serving Size: 6

Nutritional Information:

Calories - 309

Carbs - 1.5 g

Protein - 27.2 g

Fat - 21.3 g

Cook Time: 1 hour

Ingredients:

- 1 tablespoon virgin olive oil
- 1 whole chicken
- 2 rosemary springs
- 3 garlic cloves (peeled)
- 1 lemon (cut in half)
- 1 teaspoon sea salt
- 1 teaspoon black pepper

Directions:

1. Turn your oven to 450 degrees F.

2. Take your whole chicken and pat it dry using paper towels. Then rub in the olive oil. Remove the leaves from one of the springs of rosemary and scatter them over the chicken. Sprinkle the sea salt and black pepper over top. Place the other whole sprig of rosemary into the cavity of the chicken. Then add in the garlic cloves and lemon halves.

3. Place the chicken into a roasting pan and then place it into the oven. Allow the chicken to bake for 1 hour, then check that the internal temperature should be at least 165 degrees F. If the chicken begins to brown too much, cover it with foil and return it to the oven to finish cooking.

4. When the chicken has cooked to the appropriate temperature remove it from the oven. Let it rest for at least 20 minutes before carving.

5. Serve with a large side of roasted or steamed vegetables or your favorite salad.

Grilled Octopus

Octopus is a favored dish in Greece. Most American's are used to the fried version, but this Mediterranean diet approved recipe is grilled and even more satisfying to the palate. Serve this up with a side of lemon potatoes, steamed broccoli, or roasted carrots and zucchini.

Serving Size: 6

Nutritional Information:

Calories - 234

Carbs - 1.6 g

Protein - 38.8 g

Fat - 7 g

Cook Time: 15 minutes

Ingredients:

- 2 tablespoons extra virgin olive oil (plus a little extra for rubbing your grill rack)
- 3 ½ pounds fresh octopus (the head and beak should be removed)
- 1 lemon (juice)
- ½ tablespoons parsley (fresh, minced)
- 1 tablespoon peppercorns
- 1 tablespoon and 1/2 teaspoon sea salt
- ¼ teaspoon black pepper

154

You will also want a wine cork to add to the water that you will boil the octopus in. This is to help keep the octopus meat tender.

Directions:

1. Place a large pot on your stove and fill it halfway with water. Turn the heat to high and add in 1 tablespoon of sea salt, the peppercorns, and your wine cork. Allow the water to come to a boil.

2. As you wait for the water to boil, prepare your octopus. Place it on a cutting board and use a meat mallet or rolling pin to pound the octopus a few times. Begin by hitting it near the middle section then work your way out to each of the tentacles.

3. Use kitchen tongs to carefully hold each tentacle in the boiling water for a few seconds, then lift it up and dip it back into the water for another couple of seconds. Repeat this process until the tentacle begins to curl then release it into the water. Do this with each tentacle. Once all are in the water, reduce the heat to low, and allow the octopus to boil for 1 minute. Remove the tentacles from the water and set on a plate lined with paper towels to cool.

4. As the octopus cools, preheat your grill. Using an outdoor grill will give you the best results, but you can use a grilling pan on the stove as well. Turn the grill's heat to medium-high and rub a little olive oil on the grate to reduce sticking.

5. Place each of the octopus on the grill and cook for 4 minutes, turn to let the other side cook for 4 minutes as well, or until there are nice char patterns on each side.

6. Once the octopus is finished grilling transfer them to a serving platter. Cut them into pieces and drizzle the extra virgin olive oil over top. Sprinkle them with sea salt, black pepper, and fresh parsley, then squeeze the lemon over them before serving.

Baked Zucchini and Red Potatoes

This recipe is inspired by the traditional Greek dish known as *Briam*. Though it uses just a few simple ingredients, it offers irresistible flavor. This dish is filling enough to be served as your main course for dinner or can be used as a side dish. Leftovers reheat well so you can have lunch portioned out and ready for the next day too.

Serving Size: 4

Nutritional Information:

Calories - 485

Carbs - 60.4 g

Protein - 9.6 g

Fat - 26.4 g

Cook Time: 1 hour 30 minutes

Ingredients:

- ½ cup virgin olive oil
- 2 pounds red potatoes (peeled, sliced thin)
- 4 zucchinis (sliced thin)
- 4 red onions (sliced thin)
- 6 tomatoes (cut in half)
- 2 tablespoons parsley (fresh, chopped)
- 1 teaspoon oregano
- ½ teaspoon sea salt

- ½ teaspoon black pepper

Directions:

1. Begin by turning your oven to 400 degrees F so it is nice and hot when you are ready to bake your vegetables.

2. Place your 6 tomatoes into your blender and puree until you have a smooth consistency. Set to the side.

3. Take a 9 X 13-inch oven-safe baking dish (you may need to use two dishes). Layer the potatoes, zucchini, and red onions in the dish. You can alternate the layers or just layer one on top of the other. Pour the olive oil over the top. Sprinkle on the oregano, then take your tomato puree and pour it over the top of your vegetable layers. You can leave it as is or, if you want to coat everything evenly with the tomato puree you can use a spoon to mix everything. Finish by sprinkling the sea salt and black pepper over top.

4. Place the baking dish (or dishes) into your oven and bake for at least 1 hour. The vegetables should be tender and most of the liquid should be evaporated; if not bake for an additional 30 minutes.

5. Remove the dish from the oven and allow to cool just a little before serving.

Sweet and Spicy Mediterranean Chicken

This recipe is truly one of a kind. If perfectly infuses the sweet flavors of fresh pineapple with the saltiness of black olives and brings a little heat with a hint of jalapeno. This is sure to be a dish you will want to include in your frequently made meals.

Serving Size: 4

Nutritional Information:

Calories - 205

Carbs - 9.8 g

Protein - 27.3 g

Fat - 7.5 g

Cook Time: 50 minutes

Ingredients:

- 1 tablespoon virgin olive oil
- 2 chicken breasts (skinless, boneless, cut in half)
- 1 garlic clove (minced)
- ½ red onion (diced)
- ½ green pepper (diced)
- ½ red pepper (sliced)

- ½ jalapeno pepper (seeds removed, minced)

- 1 cup tomatoes (diced)

- ¼ cup pineapple (chunks)

- ¾ cup black olive (cut in half)

- ½ teaspoon cumin (ground)

- ½ teaspoon cinnamon (ground)

- 2 teaspoon cornstarch

- ½ cup chicken stock (low-sodium)

- 2 ½ teaspoon water

- ¼ teaspoon sea salt

- ½ teaspoon black pepper

Directions:

1. Start with a large skillet on your stove. Pour in the virgin olive oil. Turn the heat to medium so the oil can warm up.

2. While waiting for the oil to become hot, sprinkle your chicken breast with cumin, cinnamon, salt, and black pepper. Place the chicken into your skillet and cook for about 5 minutes. When they are a nice golden brown, flip them so they can cook for another 5 minutes.

3. Next, add in your diced red onions and minced garlic to the skillet with the chicken and cook for another 5 minutes. Flip the chicken as necessary to prevent burning.

4. Once the onions are soft, pour in your chicken stock. Add in the tomatoes, diced green pepper, minced jalapeno pepper, and black olives. Cover the skillet with a lid and allow everything to simmer for 20 minutes.

5. When there are just a few minutes left for the dish to simmer, whisk together the cornstarch and water in a small mixing dish. Then pour it into the skillet. Add in the sliced red bell pepper and simmer for another 10 minutes, or until the sauce has thicken up.

6. Once the sauce has thickened add in your pineapple chunks and cook for 5 more minutes.

7. Turn off the heat and serve with a small side of quinoa or brown rice.

Slow Cooker Fish Soup

This hearty soup incorporates a variety of Mediterranean ingredients. It will warm you up while filling you up. You can use a variety of fish for these recipes, but cod tends to hold its shape which makes it better for soup recipes. Using your slow cooker will really allow all the flavors to come for a delightfully balanced bowl of flavors.

Serving Size: 4

Nutritional Information:

Calories - 251

Carbs - 10.7 g

Protein - 43.9 g

Fat - 2.2 g

Cook Time: 5 hours

Ingredients:

- 2 cod fillets (cut into small cubes)
- 1 pound shrimp (peeled, deveined)
- ½ red onion (chopped)
- ¼ green bell pepper (chopped)
- 2 garlic cloves (minced)
- 1 cup mushrooms (diced)
- 1 cup tomatoes (diced)

162

- ¼ cup black olive (chopped)

- 2 bay leaves

- 1 teaspoon basil (dried)

- ¼ teaspoon fennel seed (crushed)

- 1 ½ cups chicken broth (low-sodium)

- ¼ cup tomato sauce (low-sodium)

- ½ cup orange juice (fresh squeezed)

- ½ cup red wine

- ¼ teaspoon black pepper

Directions:

1. Place the chopped red onions, green bell pepper, minced garlic, diced tomatoes, mushrooms, olives, bay leaves, basil, fennel seed, chicken broth, tomato sauce, orange juice, red wine, and black pepper into your slow cooker. Stir everything together then cover with your lid. Set the temperature to low and cook for 4 ½ hours.

2. Once the vegetables have become slightly tender, add the cod pieces and shrimp. Cover and cook for another 30 minutes.

3. Before serving, remove the bay leaves.

Seared Scallops

This simple sea scallop dish is easy for anyone to make. It is packed with peppers and onions and is best served on a fluffy bed of whole grain rice or quinoa. The anchovies add a subtle saltiness to the dish, so no additional salt is needed. The lemon and lime zest give the scallops and peppers a refreshing twist.

Serving Size: 4

Nutritional Information:

Calories - 332

Carbs - 12.8 g

Protein - 26.8 g

Fat - 20.1 g

Cook Time: 15 minutes

Ingredients:

- ⅓ cup virgin olive oil

- 1 pound sea scallops (large)

- 2 ounce can anchovy fillets (minced)

- 1 red onion (chopped)

- 2 garlic cloves (minced)

- 1 red bell pepper (chopped)

- 1 yellow bell pepper (chopped)

164

- 1 teaspoon lime zest

- 1 teaspoon lemon zest

- ¼ teaspoon black pepper

Directions:

1. Pour the virgin olive oil into a large skillet on your stove. Turn the heat to medium-high. Add the minced anchovies and allow them to cook for about 5 minutes. The anchovies should begin to dissolve in the heat of the oil.

2. Place your scallops into the skillet and cook for 2 minutes.

3. As the scallops cook, toss the red and yellow bell peppers, red onion, minced garlic, lime and lemon zest, and the black pepper together in a large mixing bowl. Pour this mixture into the skillet with the scallops. Allow the scallops to cook for another 2 minutes with the mixture or until the bottoms begin to turn golden brown. Then, flip the scallops and give the mixture a stir. Cook for another 4 minutes or until the scallops have turned a golden-brown color.

4. Turn off the heat and serve.

Roasted Asparagus with Poached Eggs

Roasted asparagus offers a wide range of health benefits from improving digestion to lowering blood pressure. It is filled with vitamins like vitamins A and C, folate, and is loaded with fiber. This is a simple recipe perfect for sharing and can also be used as a great breakfast dish.

Serving Size: 4

Nutritional Information:

Calories - 118

Carbs - 5.4 g

Protein - 8.1 g

Fat - 8 g

Cook Time: 20 minutes

Ingredients:

- 1 tablespoon virgin olive oil
- 4 eggs
- 1 pound asparagus (trimmed)
- ½ lemon (zest and juice)
- 1 teaspoon white vinegar (distilled)
- ½ teaspoon sea salt
- ½ teaspoon black pepper

Directions:

1. Start by turning your oven to 425 degrees F.

2. Spread the asparagus evenly on a baking sheet. Drizzle the virgin olive oil over top. Sprinkle the sea salt and black pepper over the asparagus. Place the baking sheet into your oven. Then bake for 10 minutes. Give them a toss and bake for an additional 5 minutes or until the asparagus are slightly tender.

3. As the asparagus bakes, place a large skillet on your stove. Add 3 inches of water to the skillet and turn the heat all the way up to high. Allow the water to come to a boil then add the distilled white vinegar. Reduce heat to medium-low, carefully crack the eggs one at a time into the water. Allow the eggs to cook for about 5 minutes. The whites should be firm but the yolk should still be a little soft.

4. Use a slotted spoon to transfer the eggs from the water to a plate lined with paper towels.

5. When asparagus is tender, remove from the oven. Pour the lemon juice over top and divide it into four equal portions. Place a poached egg on top of the asparagus and sprinkle the lemon zest over top.

Chapter 11:
Shopping and Meal Prep Tips With Sample Meal Plan

When it comes to making the Mediterranean diet work for you, some planning may be necessary in order for you to get better accustomed to shopping and making your meals. It can feel like a challenge when you go shopping and you are used to picking up ready-made meals and a cart full of snacks as opposed to plenty of fruits, vegetables, and grains.

Now that you have an understanding of what the Mediterranean diet is and some easy to make recipes to start out with, this chapter will show you how you can easily make the transition. The information in this chapter will provide you with helpful tips, tricks, and a sample meal plan that will set you up for success on the Mediterranean diet.

Meal Planning

Meal planning will allow you to create a shopping list that you will stick to instead of a list that you will forget and deviate from. Starting any type of diet requires some time to get used to eating the right foods. Setting aside time during your week to properly plan out your meals doesn't take much time or effort, but can make all the difference for sticking to the diet.

Meal planning is the first step you can take to ensure that you are successful on the Mediterranean diet. It is a time that you can think about what fresh fruits and vegetables you can get to incorporate into your meals. When you are meal planning, look at your local grocery ads to see what items will be on sale.

When you sit down to meal plan, first take note of what you already have on hand. What spices do you have, whole grains, frozen vegetables, and protein? Once you know what you have you can begin to create meals around those items. When creating your meals always consider how you can use items for multiple meals. Fresh blueberries can be used for breakfast and snacks. Vegetables can be used in salads, main dishes, and snacks. Consider how you will use each item throughout the week so you don't end up wasting what you buy.

When you have a plan in place, you will feel more confident about following the guidelines of the Mediterranean diet for the entire week. As you continue with the Mediterranean diet you will find that meal planning takes less time and can be a time that you include the rest of the family.

This truly follows along with the Mediterranean way of life.

Meal plan tips:

1. Make meal planning a part of your weekly schedule.

2. Have a book of go-to recipes. As you create more Mediterranean inspired meals, you want to keep track of the ones you loved and the ones you weren't so enthusiastic about. The meals you love can be kept in a cookbook or stored on your phone so you can easily look for meal ideas for the week.

3. Try something new at least once a week. In order to build up your Mediterranean recipes, you need to be trying new things to add to it. Try including new vegetables or a different spice and herb blend. By adding a simple new ingredient or changing up some of the spices and herbs, you can create an entirely new dish. This will keep your Mediterranean meals fresh and exciting!

4. Get the rest of the family involved. In order to promote a healthy lifestyle amongst all the individuals in your household, it is best to let them be a part of the whole process. Ask them what healthy snack they want for the week, if

there is any healthy dish they have been craving, or ask them for suggestions on some new things to try.

Meal Prepping

Meal prepping can help you save time in the kitchen and get to enjoying time with your friends and family. Meal prepping can be split up between two days in the week or, if you'd rather just get it all done and over with, can be done in one day. When you are meal prepping you are simply getting the ingredients ready for your recipes so you don't have to spend time washing, cutting, mincing, or measuring when you go to cook. This can make creating your meals much easier, especially if you aren't used to spending much time in the kitchen.

Meal prep tips:

1. Meal prep according to your meal plan. If you don't think you are going to use all of certain vegetables or fruits that week, you can easily store them in the freezer so they don't go bad.

2. Pick one or two days that you can dedicate to meal prepping. If possible, try to get the rest of the family involved. You can also do a majority of meal prepping while you are making a meal for dinner.

3. Invest in a wide range of airtight containers to store foods in.

4. Wash and pre-cut all your fruits and vegetables for your meals. Have them ready in containers in your refrigerator for when you are ready to cook. It is easy to do this by labeling each of the containers and what the contents are to be used for or by using color-coded containers. You can have a dry erase board on the fridge that lists what meal each color corresponds to, then all you have to do is grab the colored container you need.

5. Pre-cook whole grains so all you have to do is allow them to reheat in the cooking process.

6. Have your snacks ready to grab and go on busy days. Portion out nuts, fresh veggies, and fruit so you don't have to feel tempted to grab anything else.

7. Have your spices measured and ready to go. Mediterranean cooking tends to use a variety of spices in most recipes. If you know a recipe is going to call for a long list of spices and herbs, have them measured out and stored in a container on your counter. Then, you can simply add them all in when you are cooking.

8. Don't forget to prepare your breakfast. As mentioned, it can be incredibly easy to skip breakfast but when you have already made it, you will be less likely to skip it. You can prep oats and fresh fruit the night before or even a few days in advance.

Shopping Tips

Shopping is going to be a whole new experience for you when you transition to the Mediterranean diet, but it doesn't have to be stressful or complicated. Remember that you will be mostly buying fresh fruits and vegetables. Your local farmers market is a good place for buying produce. Go to your local farmers market first for local and in-season fruits and vegetables. It is always a great idea to talk with some of the local vendors so you have a better idea of what produce you can expect. This will help you with your meal planning as well. After getting what you can from the farmers market you can make a stop at the local butcher or seafood market if you have one. Here you can get your poultry and fish and know it is freshly caught that day. If you don't have a butcher shop or seafood market, then it is time to go to your local grocery store.

How to shop on the Mediterranean diet?

1. First, never go shopping without a list. If you don't have a list you will be more likely

to buy things you don't need or particularly want.

2. Never shop when you are hungry. If you know you are going to be out most of the day running errands and you will need to do your grocery shopping while you are out and about, have a healthy snack with you so you won't be tempted to let your stomach do the shopping.

3. When you enter your store, stick to the outside sections of the store. This is where you will find most of the fresh fruits, vegetables, poultry, fish, and dairy. Then you want to focus more on the center aisle. You obviously want to skip some aisle altogether like the chips, cookies, and candy aisles which often tend to be closer to the first and last aisles. Stick with the spice, whole grains, and olive oil aisle. Don't forget to pick up canned or dried beans too.

4. Always read labels carefully. Even if a product says 100% whole grains it is likely that many will have hidden ingredients you don't want to consume. Try to find organic products when possible.

Weekly Mediterranean Diet Meal Plan Sample

This sample meal plan utilizes a number of the recipes from the previous chapters but also includes some quick ideas for you to try. Use this as a guideline on how to set up your meals each week. You can always swap out some lunch recipes to use up leftover items from dinner earlier in the week, so you won't have to cook every single day.

Snacks should also be included in your weekly meal plan. Though no specific snack are listed for each day here are some great ideas to add:

- Fresh fruits

- Macadamia nuts, almonds, walnuts, or Brazilian nuts

- Warm pita and hummus

- Sliced vegetable with nonfat cheese like feta or mozzarella

- Trail mix of homemade granola, nuts, and dehydrated fruits

- Smoothie made with nonfat yogurt, milk, and a variety of fresh or frozen fruits and a handful of spinach.

Monday

Breakfast - Egg White Breakfast Sandwich

Lunch - Traditional hummus with fresh-cut vegetables

Dinner- Slow Cooker Moroccan Chicken

Tuesday

Breakfast - Fruits, Oats, and Yogurt Parfait

Lunch - Chicken Quinoa Salad

Dinner- Tilapia Florentine

Wednesday

Breakfast - Shakshuka

Lunch -Greek Inspired Potatoes

Dinner - White bean soup

Thursday

Breakfast - Caprese on Sourdough

Lunch - Lentil Soup

Dinner -Baked Zucchini and Red Potatoes

Friday

Breakfast - Fruits, Oats, and Yogurt Parfait

Lunch - Sliced tomatoes and cucumbers with crumbled feta and drizzled with extra virgin olive oil.

Dinner - Whole Wheat Penne with Shrimp

Saturday

Breakfast - Mediterranean Inspired Breakfast Quinoa

Lunch - Warm Cod Salad

Dinner - Asparagus With Poached eggs

Sunday

Breakfast -Eggs Florentine

Lunch - Traditional Hummus and Fresh Cut Veggies

Dinner-Seared Scallops

Recap of meal planning:

When creating your own meal plan for the week keep in mind these key tips:

1. Include as many vegetables throughout

your day as possible.

2. Enjoy whole grain with your meals

3. Include two servings of fish each week.

4. Make one meal completely vegetarian.

5. Include two poultry recipes into your week.

6. Swap out one red meat dish and sub in beans, lentils, and legumes.

7. Enjoy what you made with family and friends!

Conclusion

The Mediterranean diet is more than what you eat; it is a way of living. This diet reflects the true definition of what a diet should be. It encourages eating healthy nutritious foods, while also emphasizing the importance of physical activity and spending time with those we care about. The Mediterranean diet has been studied for decades and each time it seems a new benefit of this diet comes to light.

What Ancel Keys did when he conducted the "Seven Countries Study" was unlock the door for the whole world to see how food is negatively influencing their lives. He began a movement that may not have caught on quickly but was crucial in understanding the relationship between diet and severe health complications. Although there are studies that back up the benefits of the Mediterranean diet, and although it has been reviewed countless times and tested on various individuals with varying complications, it has yet to be the standard way of living around the world.

What needs to be done is adopting a new way of looking at food and mealtimes. Our world today stresses working harder and longer which means there is little time for enjoying meals. If we can change our perspective to see that the food we eat is what makes us more efficient and productive, then we would be able to more easily change the way we eat.

The Mediterranean diet considers various aspects of what "health" means. It does not just focus on what you eat but it also focuses on how you eat, who you eat with, and the activities you do in between eating. Each of these components can contribute to better health and a more fulfilling life. When we are lacking in any of these components, we tend to suffer from poor health, fatigue, depression and more. The Mediterranean diet was originally looked at because of its heart health benefits, but now it is clear to see that the traditional Mediterranean lifestyle from the 1950s was more than just a heart-healthy plan.

This book has introduced you to what the Mediterranean diet is. It has helped you understand that this isn't your typical diet. That instead, the Mediterranean diet is about changing into a lifestyle that will bring you better health and happiness. This book has provided you with some of the findings from scientific research that supports the diet's benefits. You have learned that the diet consists of eating plenty of fresh fruits, vegetables, and healthy fats like extra virgin olive oil. You also get to enjoy heart-healthy whole grains, brain-boosting fish and seafood and occasionally can celebrate with a nice steak dinner. This diet is not restricting you to count calories or eliminate vital food groups.

This book has helped you understand not only the benefits of this diet but has revealed effective tips and suggestions to help you transition into this type of diet. The changes can be made in small steps, because even the smallest change to shifting your diet to a more Mediterranean diet can have a whirlwind of benefits. You have learned how to swap the unhealthy foods you have been used to consuming with nutrient-dense and wholesome foods.

You now have a better understanding that this diet is not about just losing weight. It is not a diet that allows you to eat your weight in pasta, or drink equal amounts of red wine. It has shown that you can use food as a form of natural medicine to reduce and eliminate the risk of many serious health conditions. You have learned how your food directly affects the way your body functions and when it is deprived of the nutrients it needs it will not be able to perform appropriately.

The recipes in this book allow you to begin trying out delicious, flavorful, and healthy Mediterranean inspired meals. You have a number of breakfast, lunch, and dinner options that are sure to satisfy and please everyone in your home. These recipes can be your starting point in taking control of your health. In the final chapter, you were provided with an example of how to add these recipes into your weekly meal plan. This last chapter also unveiled the most effective meal planning, meal prepping, and shopping tips that will allow you to embrace the Mediterranean diet with ease.

Now that you have all this information on how you can maintain and achieve optimal health, it is up to you to decide. Will you continue to choose a life where the foods you eat leads you down a road to illness and preventable suffering? Or will you make the change now to live your life and be the healthiest and happiest version of you? All you have to do is start with one small change and then go from there. Once you begin to see the benefits from that one small choice you will be eager to try more and soon you will be living a Mediterranean lifestyle that is significantly more satisfying.

Finally, this book was designed to help you understand that diet doesn't have to make you feel like you are giving up some of your favorite foods. Instead, it allows you to find new favorites that will improve your overall health. Allow the food you enjoy today to be your medicine for your future.

References

Mediterranean Diet. (n.d.). Retrieved from https://health.usnews.com/best-diet/mediterranean-diet

Are Processed Red Meats More Unhealthy than Other Red Meats? (2019, November 22). Retrieved from http://www.center4research.org/processed-red-meats-less-healthy/

Bradley, B. (2019, January 2). How to Eat the Real Mediterranean Diet. Retrieved from https://www.mediterraneanliving.com/eat-real-mediterranean-diet/

EricT_CulinaryLore. (2018, May 28). What is the Origin of the Word Diet? Retrieved from https://culinarylore.com/food-history:origin-of-the-word-diet/

McManus, K. D. (2019, March 11). A practical guide to the Mediterranean diet. Retrieved from https://www.health.harvard.edu/blog/a-practical-guide-to-the-mediterranean-diet-2019032116194

Mediterranean diet is linked to higher muscle mass, bone density after menopause. (n.d.). Retrieved from https://www.endocrine.org/news-and-advocacy/news-room/2018/mediterranean-diet-is-linked-to-higher-muscle-mass-bone-density-after-menopause

Nutrition and Dementia: Foods That Increase Alzheimer's Risks. (2019, April 25). Retrieved from https://www.alzheimers.net/foods-that-induce-memory-loss/

Oldways Mediterranean Diet Pyramid. (n.d.). Retrieved from https://oldwayspt.org/resources/oldways-mediterranean-diet-pyramid

Pulling Ancel Keys Out from Under the Bus. (n.d.). Retrieved from https://oldwayspt.org/blog/pulling-ancel-keys-out-under-bus

Recipes. (n.d.). Retrieved from https://www.allrecipes.com/recipes

Roycor, A., & Roycor, A. (2017, February 23). Mediterranean Diet Pyramid, the Food Guide Pyramid and My Pyramid. Retrieved from http://www.mediterraneandiet.com/my-pyramid/

The Mediterranean Diet. (2020, February 12). Retrieved from https://www.helpguide.org/articles/diets/the-mediterranean-diet.htm

The Mediterranean Diet - An Up-Close Look at Its Origins in Pantelleria. (n.d.). Retrieved from https://www.todaysdietitian.com/newarchives/05011 3p28.shtml

Rockridge Press. (2013). The Mediterranean Diet for Beginners: The Complete Guide. Berkeley, CA.

Traditional Med Diet. (n.d.). Retrieved from https://oldwayspt.org/traditional-diets/mediterranean-diet/traditional-med-diet

Understanding Parkinson's. (n.d.). Retrieved from https://www.parkinson.org/understanding-parkinsons